NURSING84 BOOKS™

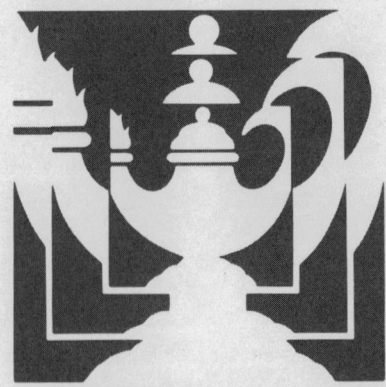

NURSING NOW™ SERIES
Shock
Hypertension
Drug Interactions
Cardiac Crises
Respiratory Emergencies
Pain

NURSING PHOTOBOOK™ SERIES
Providing Respiratory Care
Managing I.V. Therapy
Dealing with Emergencies
Giving Medications
Assessing Your Patients
Using Monitors
Providing Early Mobility
Giving Cardiac Care
Performing GI Procedures
Implementing Urologic Procedures
Controlling Infection
Ensuring Intensive Care
Coping with Neurologic Disorders
Caring for Surgical Patients
Working with Orthopedic Patients
Nursing Pediatric Patients
Helping Geriatric Patients
Attending Ob/Gyn Patients
Aiding Ambulatory Patients
Carrying Out Special Procedures

***Nursing84* DRUG HANDBOOK™**

NURSE'S CLINICAL LIBRARY™
Cardiovascular Disorders
Respiratory Disorders
Endocrine Disorders
Neurologic Disorders
Renal and Urologic Disorders

NEW NURSING SKILLBOOK™ SERIES
Giving Emergency Care Competently
Monitoring Fluid and Electrolytes Precisely
Assessing Vital Functions Accurately
Coping with Neurologic Problems Proficiently
Reading EKGs Correctly
Combatting Cardiovascular Diseases Skillfully
Nursing Critically Ill Patients Confidently
Dealing with Death and Dying

NURSE'S REFERENCE LIBRARY®
Diseases
Diagnostics
Drugs
Assessment
Procedures
Definitions
Practices
Emergencies

NURSING NOW™

DRUG INTERACTIONS

NURSING84 BOOKS™
SPRINGHOUSE CORPORATION
SPRINGHOUSE, PENNSYLVANIA

NURSING NOW™ SERIES

ADVISORY BOARD

SUSAN B. BAIRD, RN, MPH
Chief, Cancer Nursing Service
Clinical Center, National Institutes
of Health, Bethesda, Md.

LILLIAN S. BRUNNER, RN, MSN, ScD, FAAN
Consultant in Nursing,
Presbyterian–University of
Pennsylvania Medical Center,
Philadelphia

STANLEY DUDRICK, MD
Professor, Department of Surgery,
University of Texas Medical School
at Houston; St. Luke's Episcopal
Hospital, Houston

TERRI FORSHEE, RN, MS, CCRN
Visiting Lecturer, UCLA School of
Nursing; Doctoral Student,
University of Washington, Seattle

LOIS MALASANOS, RN, PhD
Professor and Dean, College of
Nursing, University of Florida,
Gainesville

ARA G. PAUL, PhD
Dean, College of Pharmacy,
University of Michigan, Ann Arbor

SPRINGHOUSE CORPORATION BOOK DIVISION

CHAIRMAN
Eugene W. Jackson

PRESIDENT
Daniel L. Cheney

VICE-PRESIDENT AND DIRECTOR
Timothy B. King

VICE-PRESIDENT,
BOOK OPERATIONS
Thomas A. Temple

VICE-PRESIDENT, PRODUCTION
AND PURCHASING
Bacil Guiley

RESEARCH DIRECTOR
Elizabeth O'Brien

PROGRAM DIRECTOR
Jean Robinson

CLINICAL DIRECTOR
Barbara McVan, RN

EDITORIAL MANAGER
Susan R. Williams

STAFF FOR THIS VOLUME

BOOK EDITOR
Katherine W. Carey

ASSOCIATE EDITORS
Holly A. Burdick
Kathy E. Goldberg
June F. Gomez
Deborah Carey Lyons

CONTRIBUTING EDITOR
Patricia R. Urosevich

CLINICAL EDITOR
Leah A. Gabriel, RN, BSN, MSN

DRUG INFORMATION MANAGER
Larry Neil Gever, RPh, PharmD

SENIOR DESIGNER
Scott M. Stephens

ASSOCIATE DESIGNER
Kathaleen Motak Singel

PRODUCTION COORDINATOR
Susan Powell-Mishler

COPY SUPERVISOR
David R. Moreau

COPY EDITORS
Dale A. Brueggemann
Diane M. Labus

CONTRIBUTING COPY EDITORS
Reni Fetterolf   David Jones
Max A. Fogel   Doris Weinstock

EDITORIAL ASSISTANTS
Ellen Johnson
Cynthia A. O'Connell
Suzanne J. Ramspacher

ART PRODUCTION MANAGER
Robert Perry

ARTISTS
Donald G. Knauss   Craig Siman
Robert S. Miele   Louise Stamper
Sandra Sanders   Robert Wieder

TYPOGRAPHY MANAGER
David C. Kosten

TYPOGRAPHY ASSISTANTS
Ethel Halle   Nancy Wirs
Diane Paluba

SENIOR PRODUCTION MANAGER
Deborah C. Meiris

PRODUCTION MANAGER
Wilbur D. Davidson

ILLUSTRATORS
Michael Adams   Bob Jones
ArtPeople   Adam Matthews
Robert Jackson   George Retseck

PHOTOGRAPHER
Paul A. Cohen

COVER PHOTO
Photographic Illustrations

CLINICAL CONSULTANTS FOR THIS VOLUME

Dawn Wade Kincaid, RN
Clinical Research Associate,
  Vanderbilt University Medical
  Center, Nashville, Tenn.

Yukie Yumibe, RN, BS, MSN
Associate Professor of Nursing,
  Pacific Lutheran University,
  Tacoma, Wash.

© 1984 by Springhouse Corporation,
1111 Bethlehem Pike, Springhouse, Pa. 19477
All rights reserved. Reproduction in whole or part by
any means whatsoever without written permission of
the publisher is prohibited by law.
Printed in the United States of America.

NN3-010684

**Library of Congress
Cataloging in Publication Data**

Main entry under title:
Drug interactions.

(Nursing now)
"Nursing84 books."
Bibliography: p.
Includes index.
1. Drug interactions. 2. Nursing.
  I. Springhouse Corporation.   II. Series:
Nursing now series.   [DNLM:
1. Drug Interactions—nurses' instruction.
QV 38 D7931]
RM302.D778   1984   615'.7045   84-5639
ISBN 0-916730-78-6

CONTENTS

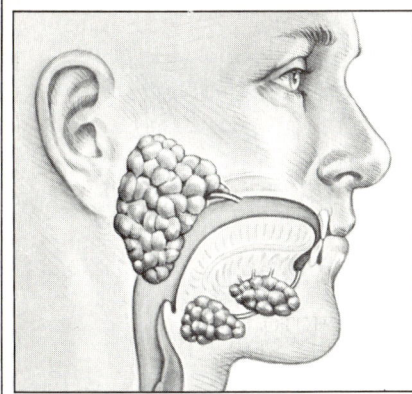
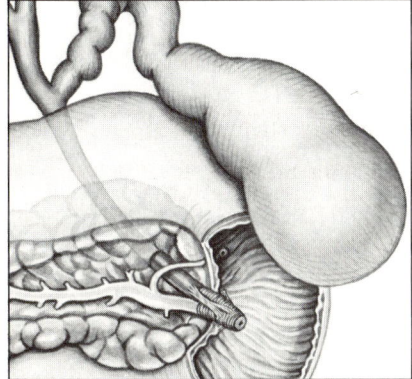
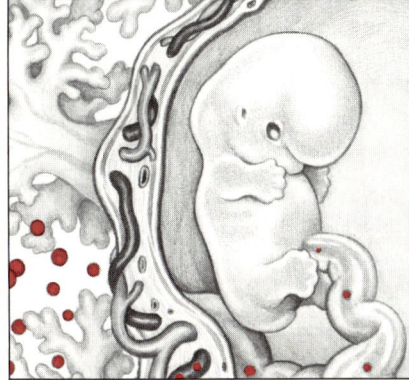
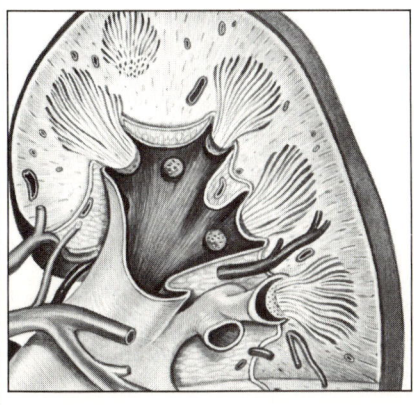

LAYING THE FOUNDATION
Leah A. Gabriel, RN, BSN, MSN

8   Your role

UNDERSTANDING DRUG ACTIONS
Judith Hopfer Deglin, RPh, PharmD
J. Ken Walters, RPh, PharmD

16   Definitions
17   Absorption
21   Distribution
24   Metabolism
26   Excretion
29   Adverse reactions
33   Allergy
35   Anaphylaxis
38   Nursing considerations
43   Generics

LEARNING ABOUT DRUG INTERACTIONS
Judith Hopfer Deglin, RPh, PharmD
J. Ken Walters, RPh, PharmD

46   General concepts
48   A.D.M.E.
54   Receptor-site action
55   Electrolytes
58   Your role

MODIFYING DRUG THERAPY
Leah A. Gabriel, RN, BSN, MSN
Barbara F. McVan, RN

62   Pregnancy
67   Pediatrics
69   Geriatrics
72   Genetics
76   Kidney disease
79   Liver disease
83   Special considerations
84   Life-style

IDENTIFYING DRUG INTERACTIONS
Judith Hopfer Deglin, RPh, PharmD
J. Ken Walters, RPh, PharmD
Dawn Wade Kincaid, RN
Yukie Yumibe, RN, BS, MSN

90   Your role
91   Analgesics
93   Anti-infectives
98   Oral anticoagulants
101   Anticonvulsants
103   Oral antidiabetics
105   Antineoplastics
106   Cardiovascular drugs
112   G.I. drugs
113   Hormones
115   Psychotherapeutic drugs
119   Miscellaneous drugs
120   Lab tests

126   Appendix
131   References and acknowledgments
132   Index

CONTRIBUTORS

At the time of publication, these contributors held the following positions:

Judith Hopfer Deglin is a consultant/clinical pharmacist at Natchauq Valley Community Health Care Services, Willimantic, Connecticut. She received her BS in pharmacy from the University of Connecticut and her doctorate from Philadelphia College of Pharmacy and Science. Dr. Deglin is a lecturer in clinical pharmacy at the University of Connecticut School of Pharmacy and a member of the American Society of Hospital Pharmacists.

Dawn Wade Kincaid is a clinical research associate at Vanderbilt University Medical Center in Nashville, Tennessee. She received her LPN from Metropolitan Nashville Vocational Training Program, Vanderbilt University, and her Associate Arts degree in nursing from the University of Tennessee in Nashville. Ms. Kincaid is a member of the Tennessee Nurses' Association and the Middle Tennessee Heart Association. In 1983, she was honored with an Outstanding Young Women of America service award.

J. Ken Walters is assistant director of pharmacy services at Hartford Hospital, Hartford Connecticut and associate clinical professor of pharmacy at the University of Connecticut School of Pharmacy in Storrs. He received his BS degree and doctorate in pharmacy from the University of Maryland School of Pharmacy in Baltimore. Dr. Walters is a member of the American Society of Hospital Pharmacists, the Connecticut Society of Hospital Pharmacists, the American Pharmaceutical Association, and the National Hospice Organization.

Yukie Yumibe is associate professor in nursing at Pacific Lutheran University, Tacoma, Washington. Ms. Yumibe received her Master of Science in nursing at Wayne State University, Detroit. She's a member of the American Nurses' Association and the Washington State Nurses' Association.

INTRODUCTION

As a busy medical/surgical nurse, you routinely care for patients who take several different drugs a day. Studies indicate that the average hospitalized patient receives from 12 to 15 drugs during his stay. And a critically or chronically ill patient could easily receive far more.

You know that a patient's risk of adverse drug reactions and interactions grows in proportion to the number of drugs he receives. To minimize his risk, you can look up the drugs you're unfamiliar with to determine the possible adverse reactions and interactions associated with them. But despite these precautions, you probably still feel uneasy when administering multiple drug therapy. We've designed this book to help you sort out this complex subject.

When you think of a drug interaction, you probably think of two or more drugs exerting an effect that alters the action of one or both drugs. And, of course, you're right. But in this book, we don't limit ourselves to discussing only interactions of this type. We'll consider a drug interaction to be any alteration in a drug's usual action in the body, regardless of the cause.

Why such a broad definition? Because the patient himself makes a unique contribution to drug action. Age, size, physical condition, and genetic factors all influence his response to any given drug combination. Any factor that affects drug action affects the patient himself—and for you, the nurse, that's the bottom line.

When you consider all the variables, drug administration takes on a bewildering complexity. That's why you'll find this book invaluable. In it, we not only detail many specific drug interactions, we examine the pharmacologic principles that should guide you when you try to anticipate possible drug interactions.

To help you meet this challenge, we focus first on drug action in your patient's body, from absorption to excretion. In addition to intended therapeutic effects, we examine how and why adverse reactions occur. Then, we discuss how interactions affecting a drug's usual action can occur at each step of the process and how to distinguish these interactions from adverse reactions.

Next, we study the patient at high risk of suffering an adverse reaction or interaction. Is he very young—or very old? Does he have a kidney or liver disorder? These and other special conditions complicate drug therapy and increase the risk of an interaction. To help you intervene appropriately, we devote an entire section to such special patients.

Beginning on page 90, we detail specific drug interactions in chart form. By consulting these charts, you can quickly find significant and well-substantiated drug interactions affecting individual drugs within major drug categories. We also provide six pages of detailed information on how drugs can alter laboratory test results.

Use this book to supplement your knowledge about drugs. We think you'll agree that it provides the practical information you've been looking for.

Barbara McVan, RN
Clinical Director

LAYING THE FOUNDATION

Administering drugs is one of your most important nursing responsibilities. And clearly, that responsibility goes far beyond knowing a drug's indications, administration routes, dosage range, and expected therapeutic effects. You also must understand how drugs interact with each other.

That's a big job. One hospital study revealed that the average hospitalized patient takes more than 13 drugs during his stay—and that taking 40 or more over several weeks is possible. The potential for adverse drug interactions is staggering.

Throughout this book, we'll provide guidelines for meeting this challenge. As always, a thorough patient assessment is the first step. Read the next few pages for key assessment considerations that can help you anticipate and avoid problems. In the rest of this section, we'll cover other nursing basics, including patient teaching and your legal responsibilities.

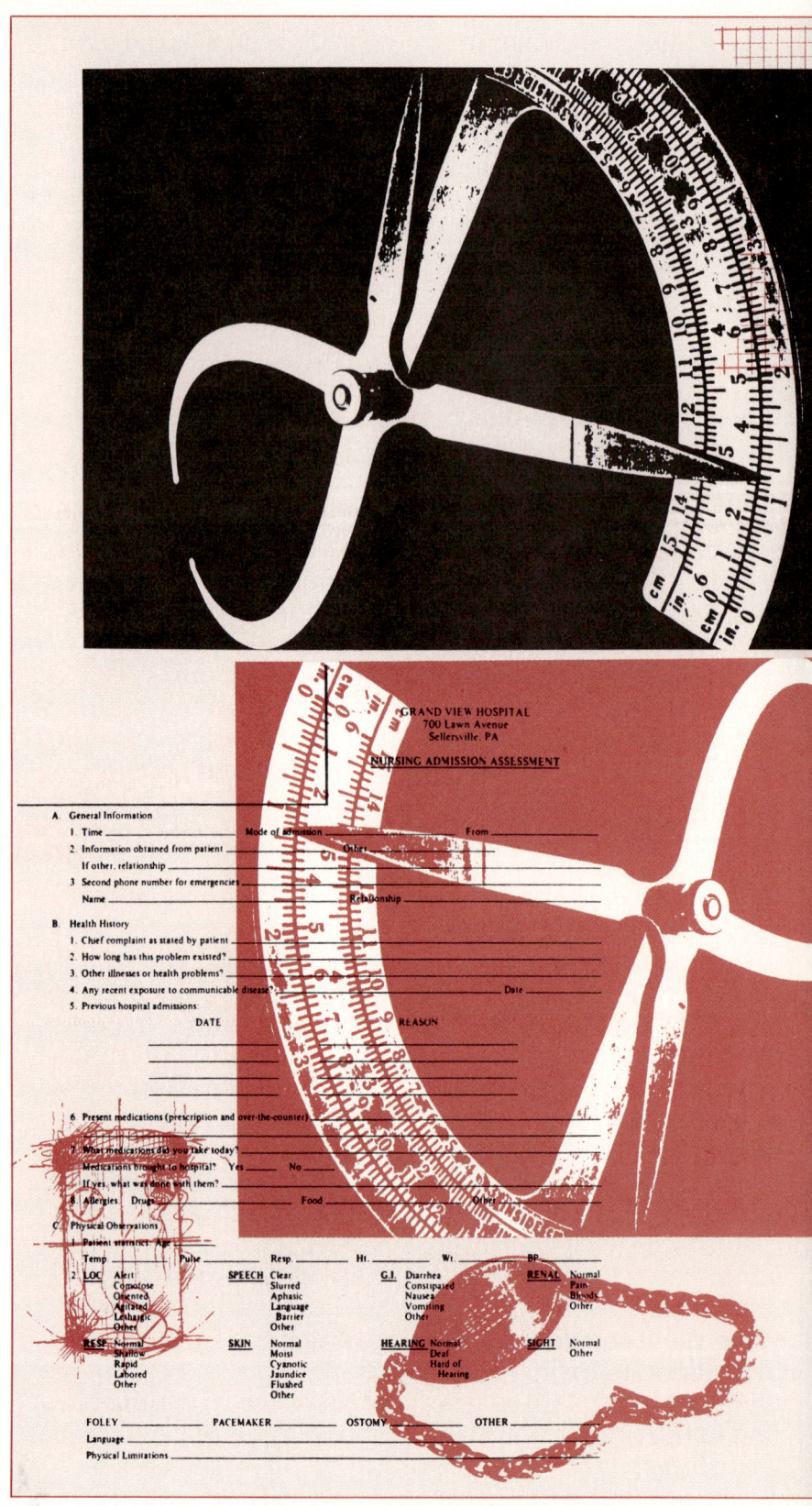

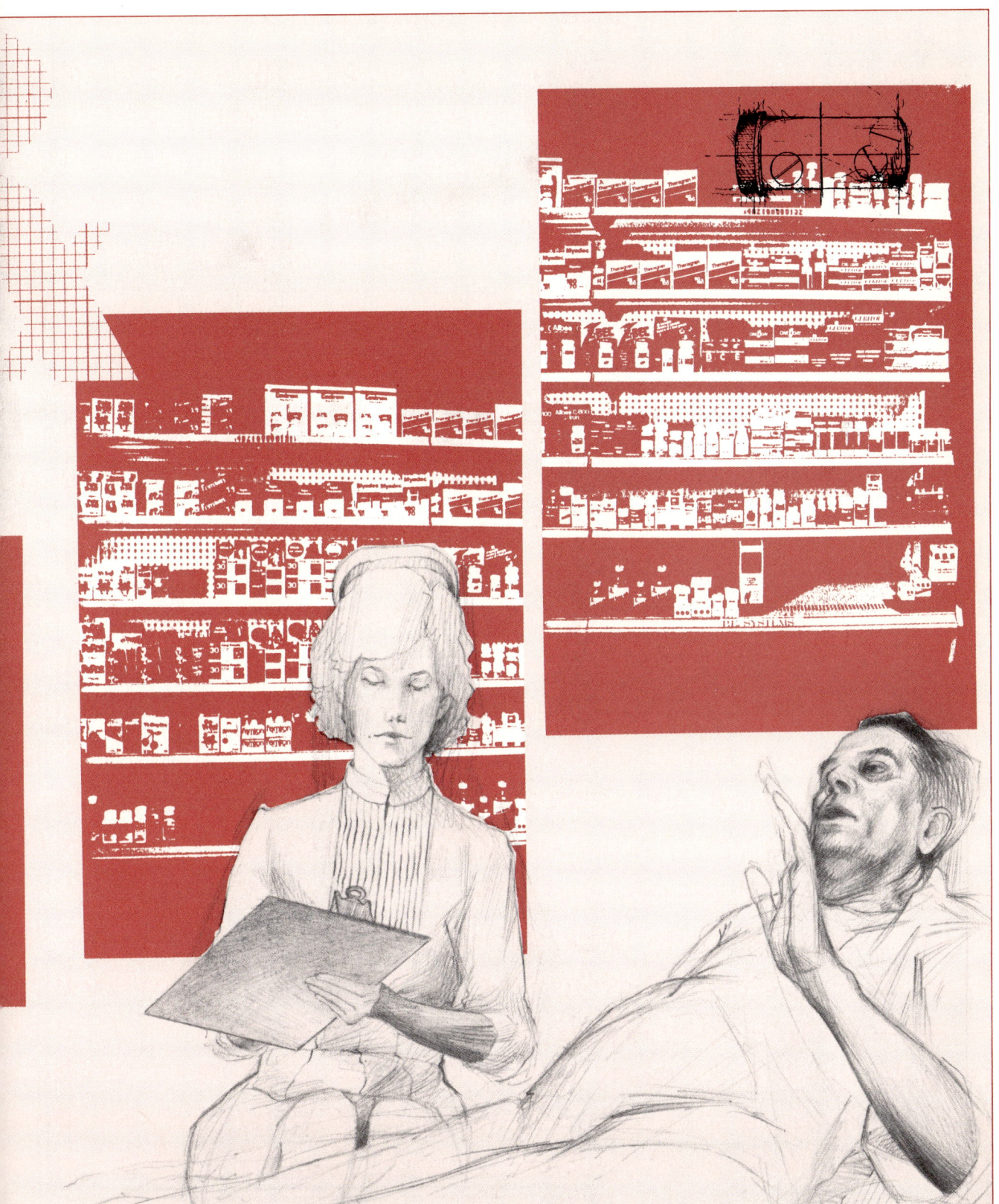

LAYING THE FOUNDATION 7

YOUR ROLE

A CASE IN POINT

You're the primary nurse caring for Edna White, a 68-year-old diabetic housewife with a fractured pelvis. From her history, you learn that she's been taking chlorpropamide (Diabinese) for several years. Her blood sugar level on admission is 180 mg/dl, so the doctor continues the Diabinese at her usual dosage.

One week after admission, Mrs. White complains of a burning sensation when she urinates; you notice her urine is cloudy. The urine specimen you send for urinalysis and culture and sensitivity reveals a urinary tract infection. You start Mrs. White on co-trimoxazole (Septra), two tablets P.O., b.i.d., as ordered.

The following morning, Mrs. White tells you that she has a headache and doesn't feel well. You notice that her breakfast is untouched, her skin is clammy, and she's having tremors. Because her signs and symptoms indicate hypoglycemia, you give her orange juice with sugar and call the laboratory for this morning's serum blood sugar level. When you learn that her level is now 60 mg/dl, you notify the doctor.

Why the dangerous drop? A drug interaction between Septra and Diabinese is to blame. The sulfa contained in Septra displaces Diabinese from protein binding sites, causing an unusually high proportion of Diabinese to circulate in the bloodstream. As a result, Diabinese has a more potent effect than intended. The consequence for your patient may be hypoglycemia.

Fortunately, Mrs. White recovers uneventfully. But her story illustrates an important point. You must anticipate possible interactions and be ready to intervene whenever a drug is added to the patient's present regimen.

CRITICAL QUESTIONS

TAKING A HISTORY

Before administering any drugs, gather pertinent information about your patient, including his medical and drug history. This information helps you assess the potential for adverse reactions and drug interactions. Use these questions as a guide.

- Why are you in the hospital? Describe your symptoms. When did they first occur? What were you doing at the time? Was the onset sudden or gradual?
- Have you ever been treated for other medical conditions; for example, hypertension or heart disease?
- Do you ever have trouble with your kidneys? Have you been urinating more or less lately? Have you ever had jaundice (or any liver problem)? How about problems with your stomach or bowels?
- Is more than one doctor treating you?
- Are you currently taking any prescribed medication? If so what is the name of each medication, the dosage, how you take it (for example, orally or by injection), and why you take it. (If he can't identify his medications, ask him to describe them.)
- Do you have your medication with you?
- Have you taken any medication today? Which ones?
- Do you take your medication as prescribed?
- Have you stopped taking prescribed medication?
- Do you ever use nonprescription (over-the-counter) medication, such as aspirin, "water" pills, weight-loss drugs, sleeping pills, cough syrup, eye drops, or laxatives? If so, what do you take, how often, and why? (Or, ask what he takes for such conditions as headache, constipation, colds, or, for a woman, menstrual pain.)
- Are you allergic to any foods, animals, insect stings, plants, vaccines, or medication? Do you have any seasonal allergies, such as hay fever? Have you ever had any other reaction to medication?
- Do you smoke (cigarettes, marijuana, pipe, or cigars)? How much do you smoke? How long have you smoked?
- Do you drink alcohol? Do you prefer beer, wine, or liquor? How often do you drink? How much?
- Do you ever use drugs for recreation?
- What's your occupation? What are your hobbies?
- Have you recently been exposed to chemicals, toxic fumes, solvents, or pesticides?
- Describe your eating habits. Do any foods upset your stomach? Do you follow any special diet?

SPECIAL ASSESSMENT CONSIDERATIONS

In addition to a patient history, your data base includes other assessment findings: among them, your patient's age and size (height, weight, and body frame). Consider these points:

Age. When a person ages, his hepatic and renal functions diminish. As a result, the rate and degree of drug metabolism and excretion slow proportionately. Because a younger person metabolizes and excretes drugs more quickly, he may require a larger dose than a geriatric patient. (We'll discuss geriatric considerations in greater detail in Section 4.)

Body size. Many drug dosages are based on the patient's weight. As a rule, a heavier patient requires a larger drug dose than a lighter patient. But to assess the relationship between your patient's size and proper drug dosage, you must consider more than his weight alone. The proportion of body fat to muscle plays a part, too. If your patient is overweight, he may actually need *smaller* doses (or longer dosage intervals), because fat stores many drugs. As a result, drugs may remain active in the body longer than they would in a very muscular patient who's the same height and weight. *Note:* Because males have a greater muscle mass to body fat ratio than females, they may require slightly larger drug doses.

To put your patient's height and weight into proper perspective, consider his body frame. See the chart at right for guidelines.

DETERMINING BODY FRAME TYPE

Suppose you have two patients who are the same height and weight. Despite their equal size, one could be overweight and one could be underweight. What makes the difference? Body frame type. Expect a large-framed person to be heavier than a small-framed person of equal height.

To determine your patient's body frame type, use this simple technique. First, measure his wrist at the narrowest circumference (between the wrist joints and the hand). Then, measure his height without shoes.

On the chart below, find his wrist measurement on the horizontal axis and his height measurement on the vertical axis. Follow each axis until they meet. The color of the block where both axes meet will tell you the patient's body frame type.

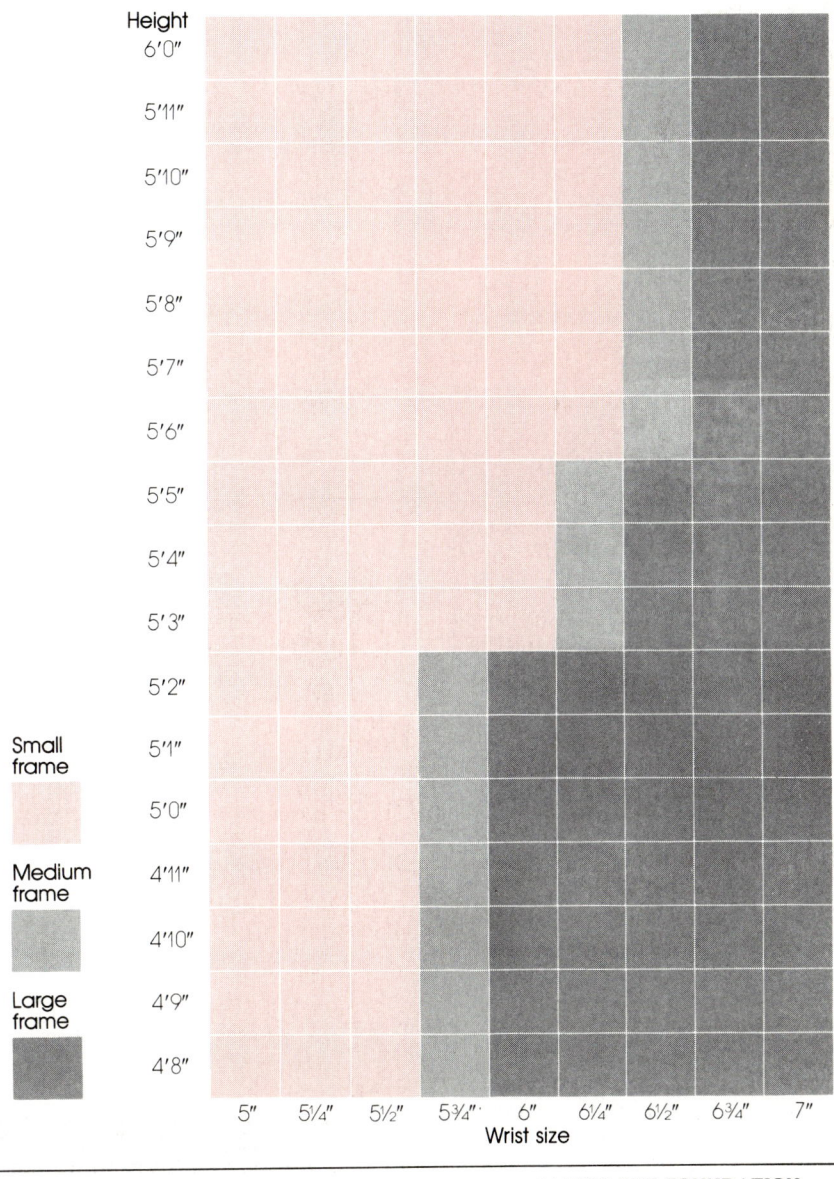

LAYING THE FOUNDATION 9

YOUR ROLE

ASSESSING FAT AND PROTEIN RESERVES

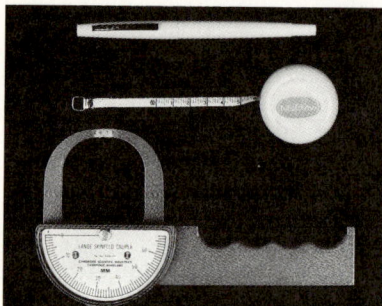

1 If your patient is undernourished, the doctor may adjust the drug dosage. Before he makes this decision, he may ask you to evaluate your patient's nutritional status by assessing his fat and protein reserves, as shown in these photos. (See the charts on page 11 to interpret your findings.)

First, gather the equipment shown here: a nonstretch centimeter tape measure, felt-tip pen, and Lange skin-fold calipers.

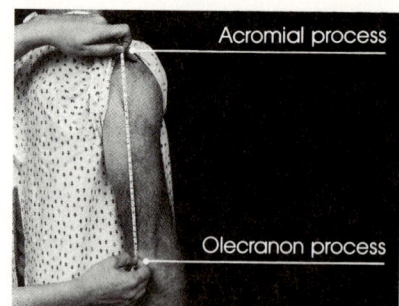

2 Explain the procedure to your patient. Then, ask him to position his nondominant upper arm at his side, as shown. Measure the distance between the tip of the scapula's acromial process and the tip of the ulna's olecranon process, as shown here. Then, locate the midpoint and mark it with the felt-tip pen.

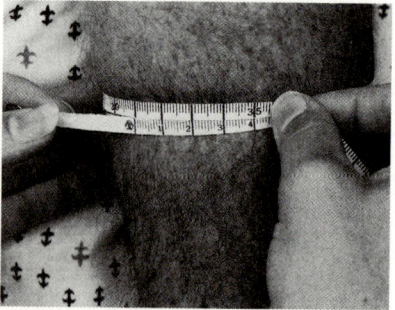

3 Measure the circumference at the midpoint. Document the result in centimeters.

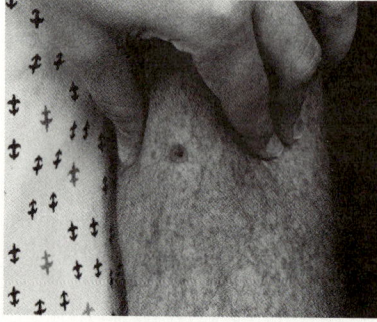

4 Now, measure your patient's triceps skin fold. First, firmly grasp a skin fold at the back of his upper arm, about 1 cm above the midpoint dot. Pull the skin fold away from the arm, so it's parallel to the arm's long axis.

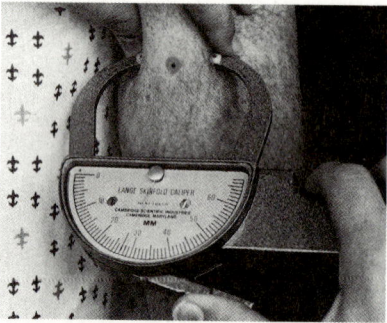

5 Then, open the calipers' jaws by pressing the lever. To measure skin-fold thickness, release the lever and let the jaws close beside the midpoint dot. Wait 2 or 3 seconds for the calipers to settle around the skin fold before taking a reading.

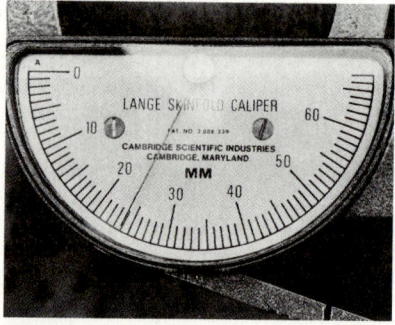

6 Round off the measurement to the nearest millimeter. Then, take two more readings (releasing the skin fold between readings) at the same site. Record the average. To calculate mid-upper-arm *muscle* circumference (indicating protein reserve), multiply the triceps skin-fold measurement (in millimeters) by 0.314; then, subtract your answer from the midarm circumference measurement (in centimeters).

10 LAYING THE FOUNDATION

INTERPRETING ARM MEASUREMENT VALUES

Compare your patient's arm measurements with the standards shown here. Keep in mind that the 100% values are standard for a patient whose weight is ideal for his height. If your patient's values are standard according to the charts, he suffers no fat or protein depletion. A value that's greater than 80% of standard indicates mild depletion; 60% to 80% of standard, moderate depletion; and less than 60%, severe depletion.

	100% (Standard)	90%	80%	70%	60%
	Triceps skin-fold measurement					
Male	12.5 mm	11.3 mm	10 mm	8.8 mm	7.5 mm
Female	16.5 mm	14.9 mm	13.2 mm	11.6 mm	9.9 mm
	Mid-upper-arm muscle circumference					
Male	25.3 cm	22.8 cm	20.2 cm	17.7 cm	15.2 cm
Female	23.2 cm	20.9 cm	18.6 cm	16.2 cm	13.9 cm

WHAT TO KNOW BEFORE YOU ADMINISTER A DRUG

When administering a medication, be sure you know all you should about its indications and contraindications, dosage, routes, compatibility with other medications and foods, therapeutic effects, and adverse effects. Here are some questions you should ask yourself.
• Why has the medication been ordered?
• Is the prescribed medication appropriate for the patient's condition? Does he have any health problems that might affect drug action?
• Is the dosage within the safe range for the drug?
• How soon will the medication take effect?
• Is the ordered route compatible with the patient's condition?
• Is the medication compatible with other medication the patient is taking? If not, tell the doctor.
• What food or other medication will affect its absorption? Knowing this, you can gauge the patient's response and help determine the cause of any adverse reactions or interactions.
• What's the medication's expected effect? If you're not sure, look it up or ask the pharmacist.
• How often will I need to check the patient after I give this medication?

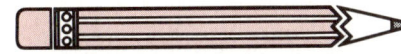

SPECIAL NOTE: Always observe the Five Rights of drug administration. When comparing the doctor's order with the patient's medication card or Kardex, check for right *name*, right *drug*, right *dose*, right *route*, and right *time and frequency*. And add a sixth right, too—right *technique*. If you notice any discrepancy, withhold the drug and check with the doctor or pharmacist.

• What adverse reactions can this medication cause? Knowing this, you can more completely gauge the patient's response to the medication.
• Does my hospital have a policy for giving this medication?
• If the medication has been ordered as needed, does the patient need it now?

YOUR ROLE IN PATIENT TEACHING

Teaching your patient about his medications is one of your basic responsibilities. With this knowledge, he's more likely to comply with therapy—and his risk of adverse drug reactions and interactions decreases. Keep these points in mind.

Teaching before discharge. As soon as your patient's well enough to be attentive, plan several brief teaching sessions. Never wait until the day of discharge to begin your teaching.

Emphasize the importance of letting you or the doctor know about *all* the medications he's currently taking, including any over-the-counter (OTC) products. Explain that some OTC medications may interact with his prescribed medication, causing adverse reactions. Or his prescribed medication may become ineffective. Warn him against taking any additional medications unless the doctor approves.

To help him remember his medications, write down the name of each one, its purpose, its dose, the correct times to take it, how to recognize adverse reactions, and which adverse reactions to report. Tape a sample tablet or capsule next to the appropriate name.

Preparing for home care. As you assess your patient's progress, stay alert for any problems he may have when he goes home. Review the following checklist:
• If your patient lives with family or friends, include them in your teaching sessions, if possible.
• If he lives alone, arrange for continuing support from a visiting nurse or social agency. Inadequate supervision may result in drug misuse, possibly leading to adverse drug interactions.
• If he can't open his medication

CONTINUED ON PAGE 12

LAYING THE FOUNDATION

YOUR ROLE

YOUR ROLE IN PATIENT TEACHING CONTINUED
bottles easily, make sure he has snap, not childproof, caps. Tell him to ask the pharmacist for snap caps in the future. *Caution:* Remind him to keep all medications out of children's reach.
• Help him work out a medication schedule based on his eating and sleeping habits. Consider setting up a medication calendar.

Alcohol is a drug that could interact with your patient's prescribed medication. Warn him against drinking alcoholic beverages or using OTC drugs containing alcohol while taking medication, unless his doctor or pharmacist approves.

• Teach him which foods to avoid and which to include in his diet.
• If necessary, refer him to your hospital's social service agency for financial help. Otherwise, he may neglect to refill his prescription or take less medication than prescribed.
• Stress the importance of taking each drug exactly as prescribed and of taking all doses prescribed. (For example, a patient taking an antibiotic may be tempted to discontinue the drug prematurely when he feels better.)
• Teach the patient how to store his medication. Caution him against mixing medications in the same container.
• Warn him against sharing his medication with anyone else.
• Urge him to inform all health professionals who care for him (including dentists and psychiatrists) about his medications.

WHAT DOES THE LAW REQUIRE?
As your role in medication administration expands, so do your legal responsibilities. At one time, nurses in the United States and Canada were allowed to administer only oral and rectal medications. Administering injectable medication was the prescribing doctor's responsibility. But times have changed. Today, nurses give subcutaneous and intramuscular injections; induce anesthesia; and start, monitor, and titrate I.V. drugs. And that's not all. With certain limitations, some states even allow nurses to prescribe drugs.

The best way to protect yourself against liabilities is to deliver quality patient care and to know your nursing rights and responsibilities in medication administration. Along with a thorough knowledge of your hospital's policy concerning medication administration, take these steps to protect yourself—and ensure patient safety.
• **Familiarize yourself with the nurse practice act from the state or province where you work.** Most nursing, medical, and pharmacy practice acts detail each profession's responsibilities and then state that anyone who carries out those responsibilities without being properly registered or licensed is breaking the law. For example, suppose you go into a drug supply cabinet, measure out a dose of a powdered drug, and put the powder into a capsule. In most states, you're practicing pharmacy without a license. As a result, you can be prosecuted and lose your license, even if no one is harmed by what you've done. In most states and Canadian provinces, practicing a licensed profession without a license is a serious offense— at least a misdemeanor.
• **Be aware of federal and state drug abuse laws.** These laws categorize drugs by how dangerous they are (forbidding the use of some and limiting the use of others) and provide for rehabilitation of drug abuse victims.
• **Know about the drugs you administer.** If you have a nursing license, you're expected to know about every drug you give. That means you're legally responsible for knowing the drug's safe dosage range, expected therapeutic effects, toxic and other adverse effects, and indications and contraindications for use.

Your responsibility doesn't end with knowing appropriate dosages. Many judges and juries now also expect nurses to know the appropriate observation interval for a patient receiving any type of medication—even if the doctor doesn't know.
• **Make sure you're giving the right drug to the right patient— and doing so correctly.** Use the familiar Five Rights system, and add a sixth checkpoint: right *technique.* (Review these and other points on page 11.)
• **Ask if you're not sure.** If you have a question about a drug order, investigate further.
—Look up the drug in a standard drug reference.
—Ask your hospital pharmacist.
—Check hospital policy for specific guidelines for giving the drug.
—Ask your charge nurse.
—Ask your nursing supervisor.
—Call the prescribing doctor.
—Ask the prescribing doctor's supervisor (service chief).
—Get in touch with hospital administration and explain your problem.
—Call your hospital's legal department.
• **Think twice before giving a drug, if you believe that doing so will harm your patient.** You may refuse to give a drug under cer-

tain circumstances; for example, if the dosage prescribed is too high, the drug is contraindicated because of possible life-threatening interactions with other drugs (including alcohol), or when you think the patient's physical condition contraindicates using the drug. When you refuse to carry out a drug order, be sure you notify your immediate supervisor, so she can make alternative arrangements (clarifying the order or assigning another nurse). Also notify the prescribing doctor, and document why you withheld the drug in an incident report.
• **Document thoroughly.** Always thoroughly document drug administration. If your patient reacts negatively to a properly administered drug, or you make an error in giving a drug, also fill out an incident report.

When documenting a medication error, chart the usual drug administration information plus the patient's reaction and any medical or nursing interventions taken to minimize harm to the patient. For the incident report, describe what happened and explain whether the cause was a nursing or prescribing error. Include the names and function of all personnel involved, and describe all actions taken after the error was discovered. Also document who was notified of the error (for example, the doctor) and the patient's responses to the error and to corrective action.

> *Can you legally give diazepam (Valium) I.V.? In some hospitals, this isn't a nursing responsibility. Make sure you know which drugs you can't give legally by checking hospital policy and your state's nurse practice act.*

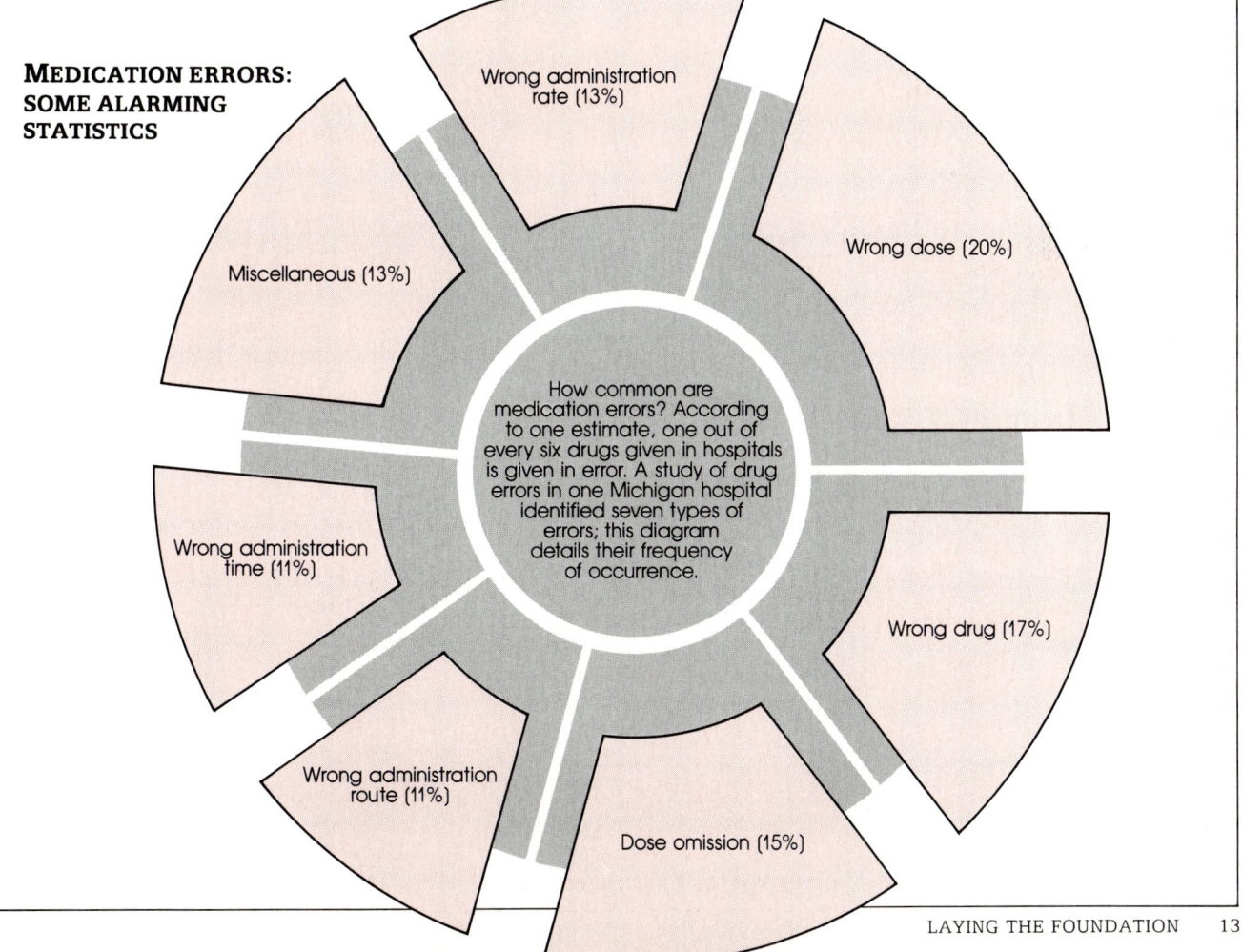

MEDICATION ERRORS: SOME ALARMING STATISTICS

How common are medication errors? According to one estimate, one out of every six drugs given in hospitals is given in error. A study of drug errors in one Michigan hospital identified seven types of errors; this diagram details their frequency of occurrence.

- Wrong administration rate (13%)
- Wrong dose (20%)
- Wrong drug (17%)
- Dose omission (15%)
- Wrong administration route (11%)
- Wrong administration time (11%)
- Miscellaneous (13%)

LAYING THE FOUNDATION 13

UNDERSTANDING DRUG ACTIONS

Whenever you administer a drug, you're starting a complex process that may continue for several hours, days, or even weeks. This process, which governs drug action in the body, includes four stages: absorption, distribution, metabolism, and excretion. What happens at each stage varies according to such factors as the drug's characteristics, the administration route, and the patient's condition. In this section, we'll discuss these and other variables in detail.

Of course, all drugs have the potential to cause adverse reactions. That's why we'll devote considerable attention to drug toxicity, allergy, and other unwanted reactions your patient may experience. In addition to examining why these reactions may occur, we'll discuss how to intervene.

Finally, we'll emphasize the administration considerations you should keep in mind to enhance drug therapy and minimize risks. Read what follows carefully.

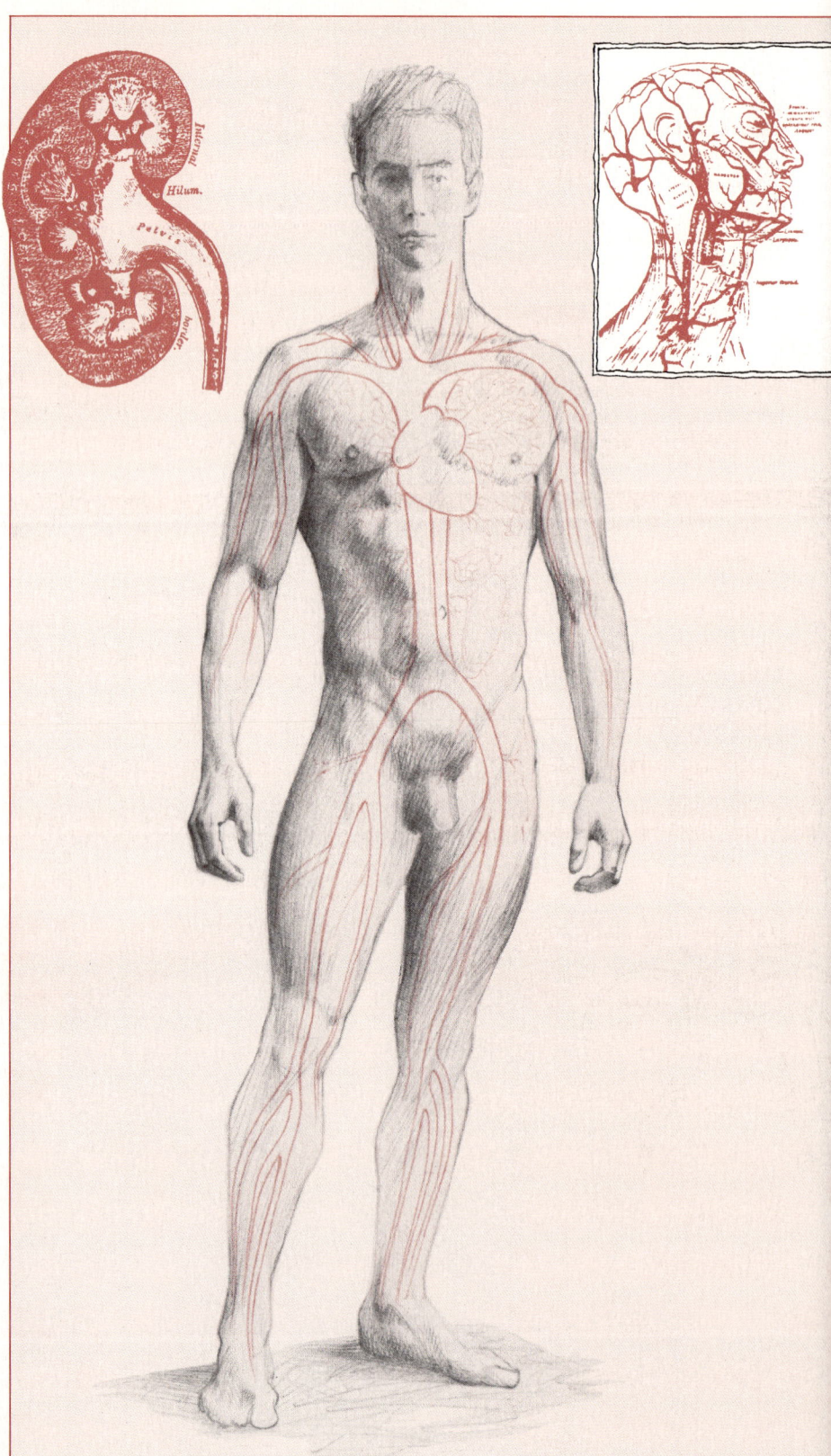

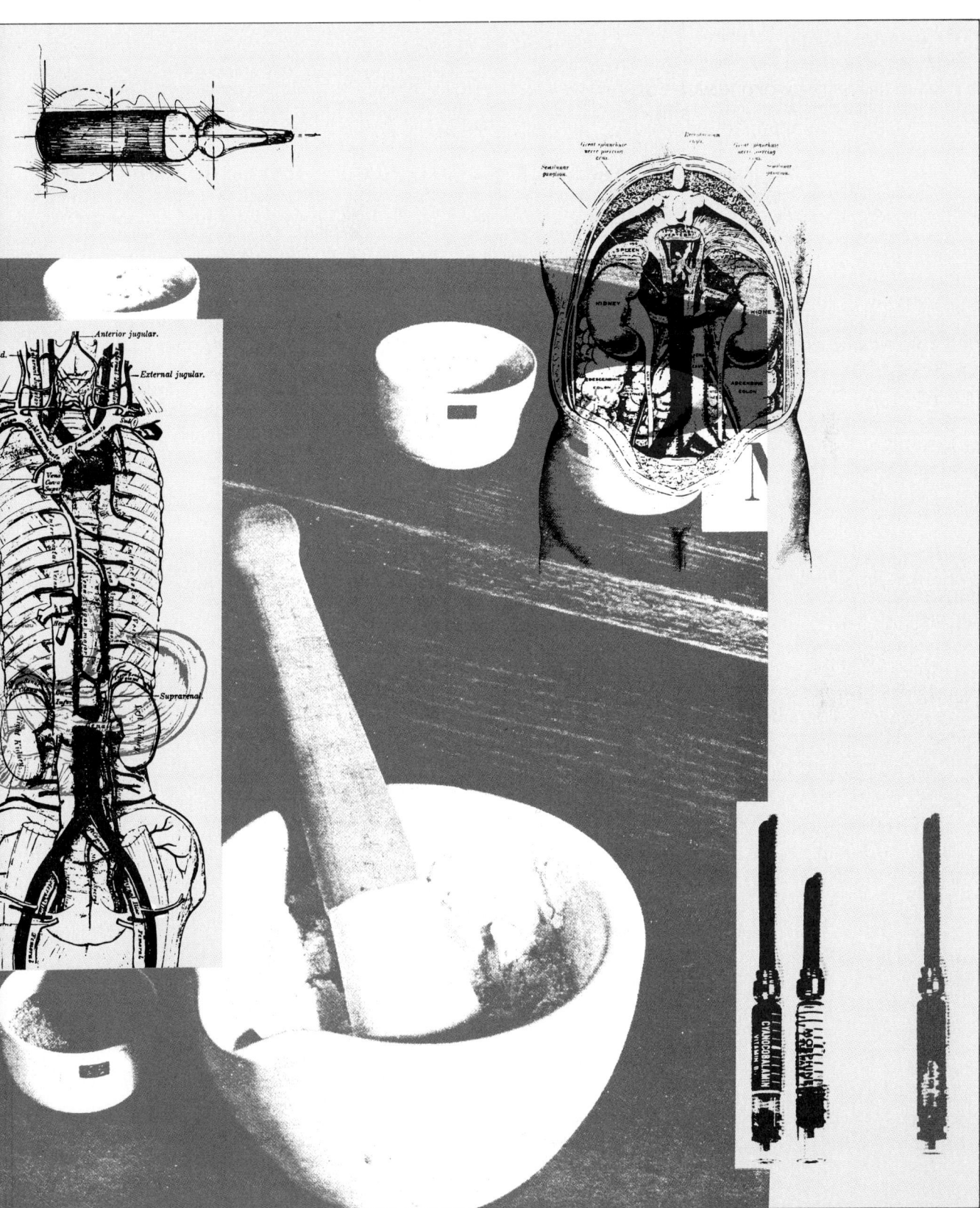

UNDERSTANDING DRUG ACTIONS 15

DEFINITIONS

Drug dynamics

Drugs are invaluable tools for the job of maintaining or improving health—but they are simply tools, not magic wands. And, like other tools, they can do more harm than good if handled improperly.

In this section, we'll explore what can go wrong, and how you can reduce the risks of undesirable drug interactions and other adverse reactions. But first, we'll review drug action in the body, from absorption to excretion.

Take a moment to review the terms in the following glossary. You'll be seeing them again throughout this section.

A glossary of terms

Acid. Any compound that can give up a hydrogen ion (proton) in a chemical reaction; an acid can combine with a base to form a salt.

Addition. Two drugs acting simultaneously by the same mechanism; their combined effect equals the sum of the two drugs' individual effects.

Adverse reaction. Any undesirable drug effect. Compare with *side effect*, page 17.

Agonist. A drug that mimics the activity of a naturally occurring substance or stimulates a receptor.

Allergy. Hypersensitivity resulting from exposure to an antigen.

Anaphylaxis. A severe, life-threatening allergic reaction characterized by release of histamine and other vasoactive substances. Response includes generalized itching, hyperemia, angioedema, vascular collapse, bronchospasm, and shock.

Antagonist. A drug that blocks the activity of another drug or of some naturally occurring substance.

Antibody. An immunoglobulin produced by lymphoid tissues in response to bacteria, viruses, or other antigenic substances.

Antigen. Any substance (usually a protein) provoking an immune response by causing the formation of an antibody specific for that substance.

Base. A substance that can accept hydrogen ions from any solution and combine with them in a chemical reaction; a base can combine with an acid to form a salt.

Bioavailability. The availability of a drug (or other substance) for activity in the target tissue.

Bioequivalent. Of or pertaining to a drug that has the same effect in the body as another drug, usually one nearly identical in its chemical formation.

Biotransformation. The chemical changes a substance undergoes in the body, as by the action of enzymes; metabolism.

Diffusion. The process by which ions and molecules move from an area of greater concentration to an area of lesser concentration, resulting in an even distribution of molecules.

Dissolution. The dissolving of one substance into another.

Enzyme. A protein produced by living cells that catalyzes chemical reactions in organic matter.

Enzyme induction. Stimulation of drug-metabolizing enzymes by a drug or other substance.

Free drug. Drug that's not bound to protein; it's therefore available to act on receptors.

Generic name. A nonproprietary name assigned to a drug; usually derived from its chemical name.

Half-life. The time required for the body to eliminate one half of the amount of drug in the bloodstream by regular physiological processes.

Hypersensitivity. An abnormal condition characterized by an excessive response to a particular stimulus, such as an antigen.

Idiosyncrasy. Hypersensitivity to a drug (often on first exposure) that is uncharacteristic of usual dose-related or allergenic responses to the drug; idiosyncrasy is not characterized by antibody formation.

Ion. An atom or molecule with a positive or negative electrical charge.

Ionize. To become electrically charged.

Lipid. Fat; this organic substance is insoluble in water.

Metabolite. A substance produced by metabolism; the product of a drug after it's been broken down or metabolized.

ABSORPTION

Polypharmacy. Concurrent administration of several drugs.

Protein binding. The process that combines a drug molecule to a protein molecule, thereby preventing the drug molecule from attaching to a receptor.

Receptor. A specialized area on the surface of a cell that can combine with particular drugs.

Side effect. A usually unwanted but predictable drug effect; the term is sometimes used interchangeably with *adverse reaction*, the preferred term in most situations.

Substrate. The substance acted upon by an enzyme.

Synergism. Two drugs working simultaneously and enhancing each other's effects, so that their combined effect is greater than the sum of the two individual effects.

Tachyphylaxis. A phenomenon in which repeated administration of a drug results in marked and rapid tolerance to the drug in a short period of time; as a result, the drug becomes ineffective.

Teratogen. Any drug (or other substance or agent) that causes abnormal fetal development.

Therapeutic index. The ratio of a drug's toxic dose to its minimally effective dose.

Tolerance. Decreased response to repeated doses of a drug.

Toxicity. A condition resulting from too much of a drug or other substance, causing toxic (poisonous) effects.

GETTING ACQUAINTED WITH PHARMACOKINETICS

Pharmacokinetics. The word sounds intimidating. But it simply refers to the four basic processes a drug undergoes after it enters your patient's body: absorption, distribution, metabolism, and excretion.

Within this framework, the composition of each drug determines how and where it's absorbed, to what areas it's distributed, how completely and at which sites it's metabolized, and how quickly it's excreted. Of course dosage form and amount, the patient's condition, and other therapeutic and environmental factors can affect any drug's progress in the human body.

By becoming familiar with pharmacokinetics, you'll be able to spot potential sources of trouble. For example, if your patient has severe diarrhea, you'll know that an oral medication may not remain in his gastrointestinal tract long enough to be fully absorbed.

Once you're aware of the possibility of problems, you'll anticipate them—and be ready to start corrective measures sooner. And your awareness of the journey individual drugs take will also help you to understand the ways one drug may affect another—as we'll discuss thoroughly in later sections of this book. For now, let's begin by discussing the absorption process.

ABSORPTION: THE FIRST STEP

Absorption, the first process any drug undergoes, brings the drug from the administration site into the circulatory system.

When a drug is administered I.V., its absorption is immediate and complete; the drug is 100% bioavailable. But a drug given by any other route has to penetrate one or more lipid cell-membrane barriers before it reaches the circulatory system. (For orally administered drugs, as you'll learn, the absorption process is particularly complex.)

CONTINUED ON PAGE 18

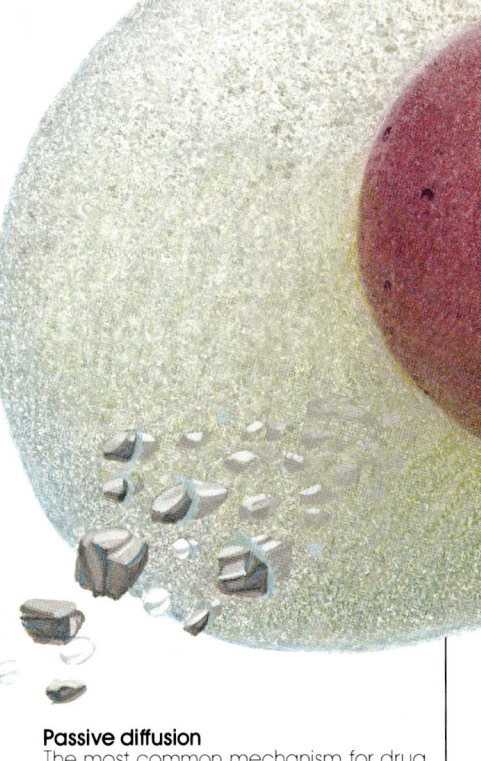

Passive diffusion
The most common mechanism for drug absorption by cells, this process doesn't require any energy expenditure.

UNDERSTANDING DRUG ACTIONS 17

ABSORPTION

ABSORPTION: THE FIRST STEP CONTINUED

How does a drug cross these cell barriers? By one of four transport mechanisms:

Passive diffusion is by far the most common and important transport mechanism. When a drug is present in greater concentration in the GI tract than in the bloodstream, a *concentration gradient* exists. If the drug is lipid-soluble (as most drugs are), the concentration gradient alone transports the drug through the membrane and into the bloodstream, with no energy expenditure required, until drug concentrations on both sides of the membrane equalize.

Facilitated diffusion also operates by means of the concentration gradient, but it allows substances with low lipid solubility to penetrate cell membranes by combining these substances with carrier substances. Like passive diffusion, this process expends no energy.

Active transport works against the normal concentration gradient, so it requires energy. In active transport, the drug combines with a carrier that takes it from a low-concentration area to a high-concentration area.

Active transport delivers some ions, sugars, and other naturally occurring substances to cells. The only drugs known to be absorbed by this method are ones that closely resemble these natural substances.

Pinocytosis is a form of active transport that occurs when the cell membrane forms a small indentation and engulfs a droplet of fluid. Although newborns are capable of absorbing several substances by pinocytosis, adults absorb only a few substances this way.

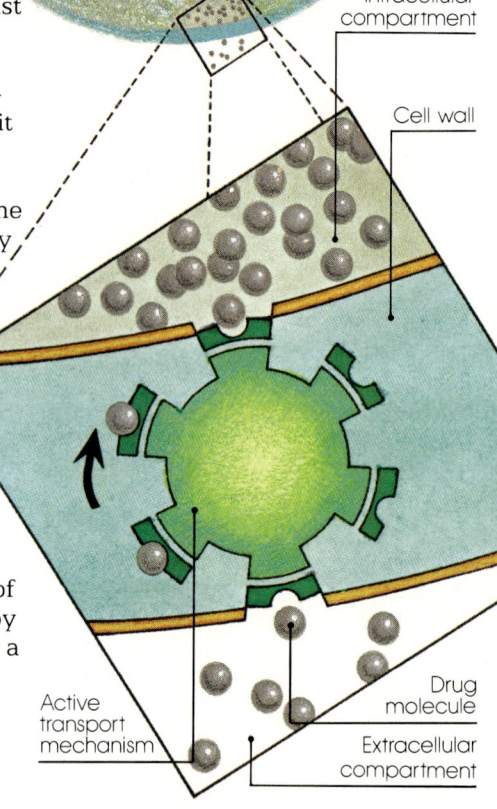

Active transport
In this conceptual illustration, an active transport mechanism allows drug molecules to move against the concentration gradient.

Pinocytosis
Only a few drug types can be engulfed and absorbed by this active transport process.

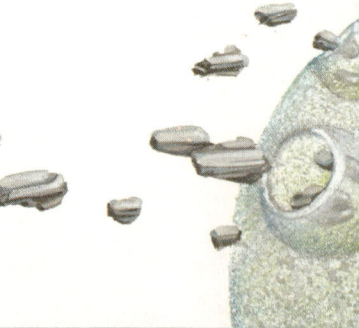

Facilitated diffusion
This illustration represents how drug molecules move from a high-concentration area (in this case, outside the cell) to a low-concentration area (inside the cell), with the help of a carrier mechanism.

WHAT AFFECTS ORAL DRUG ABSORPTION?

Both patient condition and drug composition can influence the way an oral drug is absorbed in the GI tract. The chart below provides a quick summary of the major influences.

PATIENT CONDITIONS

Factor	Effect
Rate of gastric emptying	Increased gastric emptying speeds the absorption rate of all but poorly or erratically absorbed drugs.
GI motility	In most cases, increased motility speeds the drug absorption rate. However, with very rapid motility, the total amount of drug absorbed may decrease.
pH of GI tract	A changing pH has variable effects, depending on the drug. Certain drugs require a specific pH for optimal absorption.
Presence of food in GI tract	Food slows absorption rate and may prevent drug absorption in some cases.
Presence of antacids in GI tract	Antacids alter absorption by changing the pH: they decrease absorption of most acidic drugs; increase absorption of basic drugs. Antacids also react with some drugs, forming complexes that are not well absorbed.
Fluid intake	Fluid intake with medication prevents drugs from lodging in the esophagus, promotes dissolution, and enhances drug passage to the small intestine. As a result, absorption increases.
Blood flow	Decreased blood flow to the GI tract decreases absorption.

DRUG COMPOSITION

Factor	Effect
Drug form	Liquid drug forms are absorbed more quickly than solid forms, because drug dissolution has already occurred.
Amount and type of inert ingredients	Disintegrants speed absorption; buffers may slow absorption.
Enteric coating	A coating prevents drug dissolution in the stomach, which delays absorption.

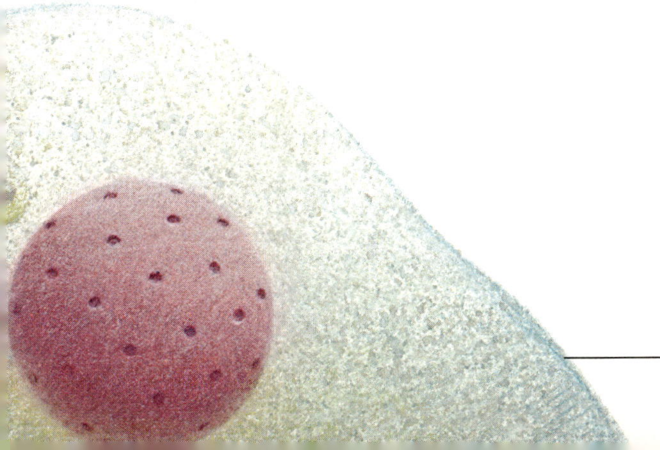

LEARNING ABOUT G.I. ABSORPTION

Your patient's probably taking most of his medications in oral form, which means that they're absorbed from the GI tract. This route has some distinct disadvantages. For example, GI absorption is slower and less complete than absorption from other sites (except rectal) because of first-pass metabolism (see page 25) and other factors. And, as the chart at left shows, patient condition and drug composition affect absorption from the GI tract, too. For more details on the factors affecting absorption of orally administered drugs, read the following information closely.

Breaking down for action. Drugs can't be absorbed until they undergo dissolution. When your patient swallows a tablet or capsule, his GI fluids must dissolve the solid medication before the drug can begin to act.

To aid dissolution, most tablet formulations include a disintegrating agent, such as starch or methylcellulose. The agent causes the tablet to swell and break into particles. This breakup creates increased surface area for GI fluid to act upon, so the drug can be absorbed more quickly. (Crushing a tablet speeds the process further. For guidelines on when you can safely crush a tablet, see page 42.)

Absorption influences. After the drug has been dissolved, it's ready to be absorbed. But absorption doesn't happen at the same rate for every drug. As a rule, the more lipid-soluble a drug is, the more easily it can be absorbed. Since mucosa in the GI tract are lipid membranes, lipid-soluble substances pass more readily through them. Water-soluble drugs, on the other hand, penetrate more slowly.

CONTINUED ON PAGE 20

ABSORPTION

LEARNING ABOUT G.I. ABSORPTION CONTINUED

Although the GI tract is a single entity, the stomach, small intestine, and large intestine each absorb drugs somewhat differently. In general, the small intestine absorbs the greatest amount of drug, the stomach less, and the large intestine the least.

Why the difference? Four factors influence absorption from these sites:
• surface area
• environmental pH
• blood supply
• emptying time.

Each site is influenced by a unique combination of these factors, so the process isn't uniform. Let's look at how each factor affects absorption.

Surface area. The small intestine presents the greatest amount of surface area for drug absorption: not just the intestinal walls, but also the thousands of villi projecting from them (see the illustration above). The amount of drug that can be absorbed at any moment depends directly on the amount of surface area available for it to be absorbed from; thus, the small intestine may absorb more drug than the stomach or the large intestine.

Environmental pH. Chemical environment varies along the length of the GI tract. Stomach fluid, which has a pH of about 2, is highly acidic. Intestinal fluid, in contrast, becomes increasingly alkaline, with a pH range from 5 or 6 in the duodenum to 8 in the terminal ileum. This pH variation affects ionization (electrical charge) of drugs, which, in turn, affects lipid solubility as drugs progress through the GI tract.

Like all lipid membranes, the intestinal mucosa repel ionized drug molecules. In the low-pH (acidic) environment of the stomach, weak-base drugs like quini-

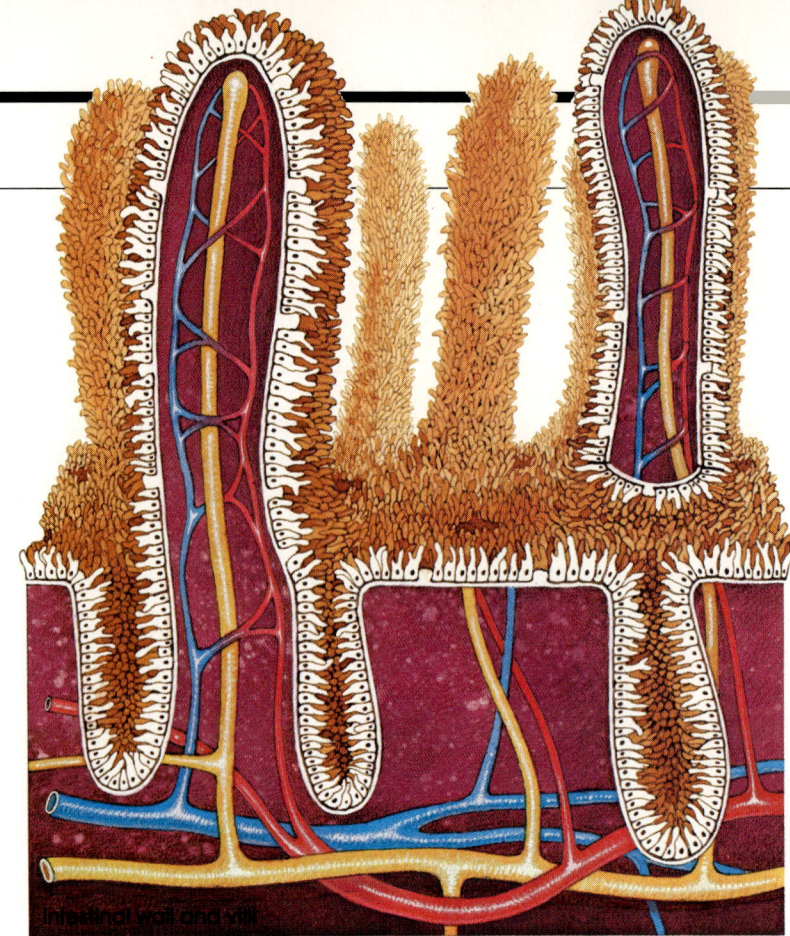

Intestinal villi—tiny, fingerlike projections from the intestinal wall—increase the GI tract's surface area approximately eight times. As shown in the cross sections, each villus contains a network of veins, arteries, and lymph channels. In addition, each is covered with microvilli, which further increase intestinal surface area.

dine are highly ionized and poorly absorbed. When a weak base reaches the more alkaline intestine, it becomes nonionized and, therefore, lipid-soluble. It can then penetrate cell membranes.

For weak acids like aspirin, the situation reverses. In the acidic stomach, aspirin is nonionized and lipid-soluble, so it's absorbed quickly. But aspirin that reaches the intestine becomes ionized, so its molecules aren't absorbed as quickly as they were in the stomach. However, because the small intestine has such a large surface area, it will absorb aspirin that reaches it.

Blood supply. The better the blood supply to an area where a drug is being absorbed, the greater the concentration gradient and the faster the absorption rate. The small intestine's normally excellent blood supply is yet another reason why most absorption occurs there. Poor blood flow, whatever its cause, may make absorption unpredictable.

Emptying time. The length of time a substance remains in any part of the GI tract can affect both the rate and amount of absorption. In most cases, slower emptying time and intestinal motility decrease the *rate* of absorption because the drug takes longer to reach the small intestine, the main absorption site for most drugs.

In a few cases, though—if the drug in question is poorly soluble or erratically absorbed—longer emptying time may increase the

20 UNDERSTANDING DRUG ACTIONS

DISTRIBUTION

amount of drug absorbed, in spite of the slower rate. When the drug reaches the small intestine, it remains there longer, so it can be better absorbed.

Food in the stomach may slow emptying time and delay a drug's progress toward the small intestine. Diarrhea and other conditions that increase intestinal motility may rush the drug through too quickly for complete absorption. (This is a particular problem with sustained-release preparations, which must remain in the small intestine for a relatively long period for complete absorption to occur.)

Gastrointestinal pH
pH varies throughout the GI tract, as shown here. Weak-acid drugs are absorbed best in the acidic stomach; weak-base drugs are absorbed best in the alkaline small intestine.

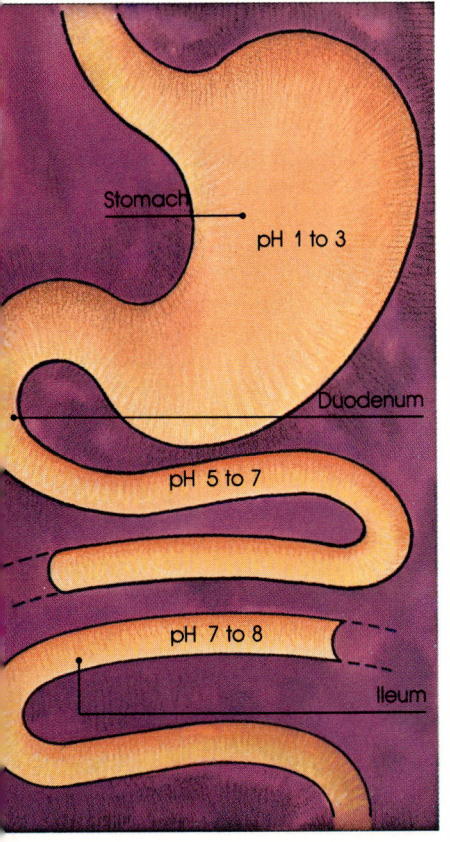

UNDERSTANDING DISTRIBUTION

Distribution is the second step in a drug's progress through the body. As drug molecules are absorbed into the bloodstream, some become bound to plasma proteins or red blood cells while others remain free. Both bound and free molecules are carried to the body's fluid compartments and tissues, where free drug molecules eventually combine with receptors to take effect.

Traveling time. How soon an absorbed drug reaches its target area depends on the area's blood supply. Drug molecules quickly reach highly vascular organs, such as the heart, liver, and kidneys. They take longer to reach less vascular areas (muscle, fat, and skin, for example).

For some drugs, the distribution process slows when they encounter certain types of membranes. Digoxin and gentamicin, for instance, have difficulty penetrating fatty tissue. And many drugs can't cross the blood-brain barrier (see page 23).

Apparent V_D. Because of their chemical makeup, some drugs distribute out of plasma into extravascular (interstitial and intracellular) fluid, thereby reaching a greater amount of total body fluid. For these drugs, the *apparent volume of distribution* (V_D) is larger, meaning that a relatively high proportion of drug becomes concentrated in extravascular fluid. V_D is a term that describes the fluid volume a drug *appears* to distribute into, although it doesn't really correlate with any physiologic volume or space.

The greater a drug's V_D, the more it's diluted. Standard dosage calculations for drugs take this into account. But your patient's condition may call for more or less than the standard dosage. A patient with edema, for instance, has more body fluid than normal. If this patient takes a drug with a high V_D (propranolol, for instance), he may need a larger-than-usual dose to receive a therapeutic effect. A dehydrated patient, on the other hand, may experience toxic effects from a standard dose.

RECEPTOR SITES: WHERE THE ACTION IS

Receptors are the part of the cell membrane that interacts with a drug to produce a therapeutic effect. Most receptors are proteins or nucleic acids. However, enzymes, lipids, and carbohydrate residues can also act as receptors.

Besides combining with drugs, receptors combine with the naturally produced chemicals—hormones and neurotransmitters—that regulate body processes. In fact, most drugs work by mimicking (or, in some cases, blocking) the action of the hormone or other chemical that normally attaches to the receptor site.

Affinity. A drug's ability to bind with a receptor is called its *affinity* for the receptor. Affinity depends on the molecular structure of both drug and receptor. These qualities permit a drug to fit with some receptors but not others.

Drugs can be *specific* or *selective* for receptors. A drug is *specific* if it interacts with only one receptor type. If the receptor type is found at several locations throughout the body, the drug can interact at each location. A drug is *selective* if it produces an effect on a receptor type at only one location, without affecting

CONTINUED ON PAGE 22

UNDERSTANDING DRUG ACTIONS

DISTRIBUTION

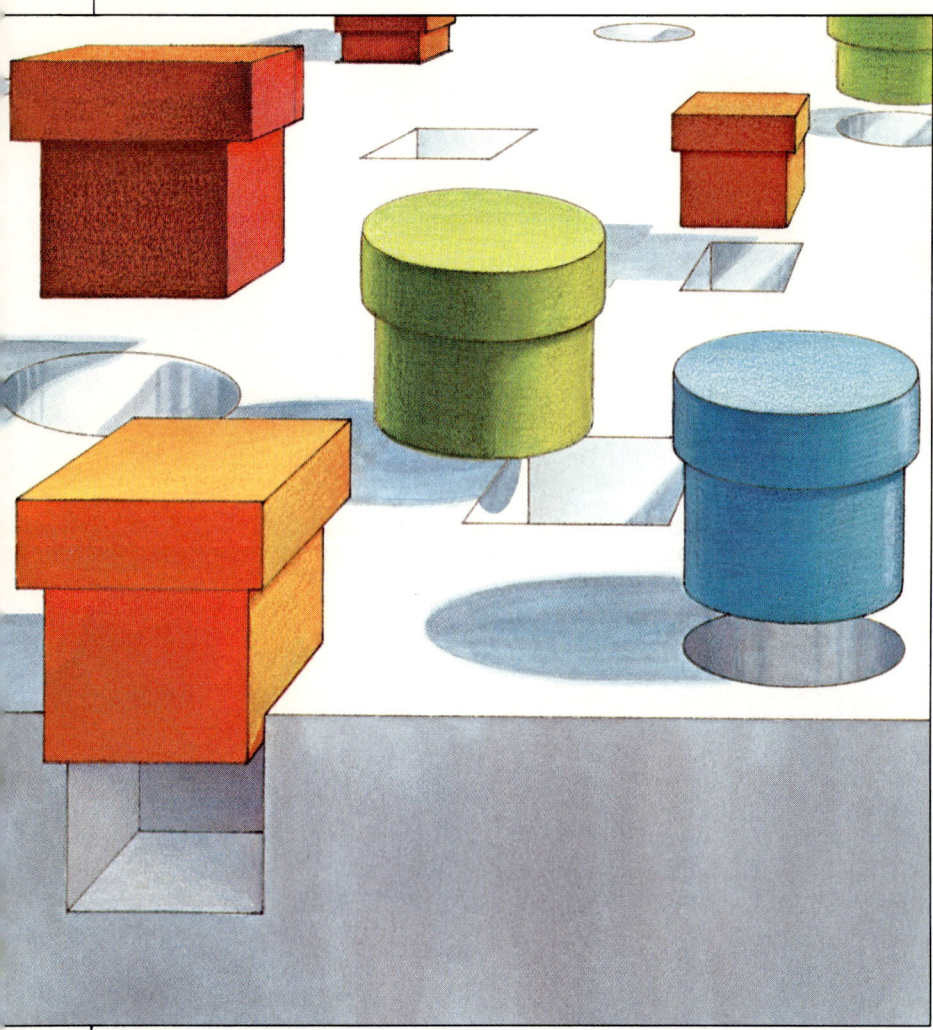

Binding at receptor sites
Just as round pegs fit only into round holes, drug molecules bind only with receptors that have the right chemical fit. This illustration represents drug molecules combining with their corresponding receptors.

A CLOSER LOOK AT PROTEIN BINDING

Not all absorbed drug molecules rush straight to receptor sites. As a drug enters the bloodstream, some of its molecules bind to plasma proteins (in most cases, to albumin) or to red blood cells.

The percentage of protein binding varies among drugs (see page 23 for examples). But whatever the drug, only its free molecules can attach to receptors and exert a pharmacologic effect. Bound molecules remain inactive, because the plasma proteins (or red blood cells) to which they're bound are too large to penetrate capillary membranes and reach receptors.

Such inactivity usually isn't permanent. In fact, the more extensively a drug is bound, the greater its duration of action in the body can be. The plasma proteins act as a storage area for the drug (something muscle, fat, and other body tissues also do for some drugs). As the body metabolizes and excretes the free drug, the plasma proteins release enough bound drug to keep the bound/unbound ratio constant. The continuing gradual release maintains therapeutic drug levels in the body.

Any disturbance of the bound/unbound ratio can have serious consequences. If, for instance, a patient begins a second drug that normally binds to the same proteins as another drug he's taking, neither drug can bind fully. As a result, a higher-than-normal percentage of at least one drug is free to distribute through the body and attach to receptor sites. In some circumstances, the patient might as well have taken an overdose.

This type of interaction occurs when the patient takes warfarin sodium (Coumadin) and phenylbutazone. Because phenylbutazone displaces warfarin, more

RECEPTOR SITES: WHERE THE ACTION IS CONTINUED

others of the same type. Some beta blockers, for example, selectively affect beta₁ sites; others, beta₂ sites.

Agonists and antagonists. Drugs can be either *agonists* or *antagonists* in the way they work at a receptor site. An *agonist* mimics the activity of the hormone or other naturally produced chemical that normally binds to the receptor site. The agonist's affinity for the receptor and its concentration at the site determine the strength of response to the stimulus it provides.

An *antagonist* blocks the action of the agonist drug or of the natural substance that normally acts on the receptor. The blocking effect of a *competitive antagonist* can be cancelled out with a higher dose of the agonist it's blocking. A *noncompetitive antagonist* inactivates the receptor rather than the agonist, so an agonist can't reverse its action, regardless of the dosage.

22 UNDERSTANDING DRUG ACTIONS

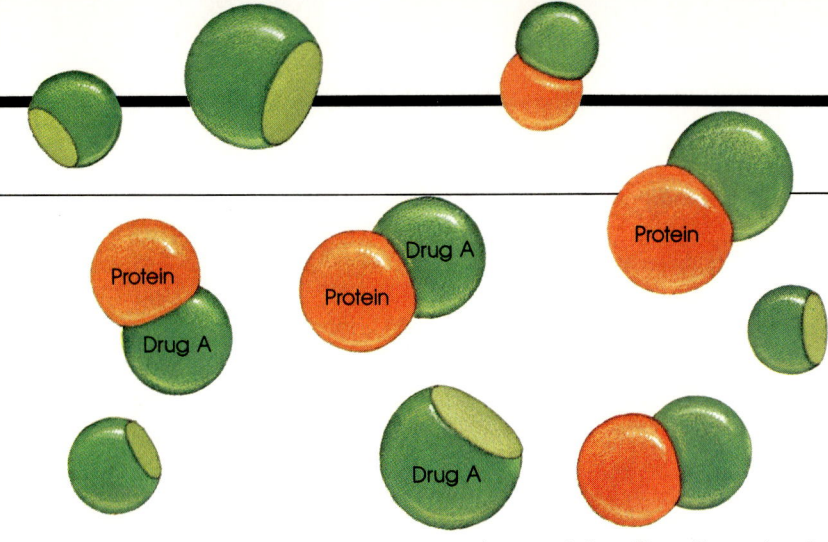

Protein binding. When a drug enters the bloodstream, some drug molecules bind to proteins; others remain free. The illustration above shows both bound and unbound molecules of an absorbed drug (Drug A).

A second drug (Drug B) entering the bloodstream may compete with Drug A for protein-binding sites (see illustration below). If some of Drug A is displaced, a greater-than-usual amount is free and therefore available to bind with receptor sites.

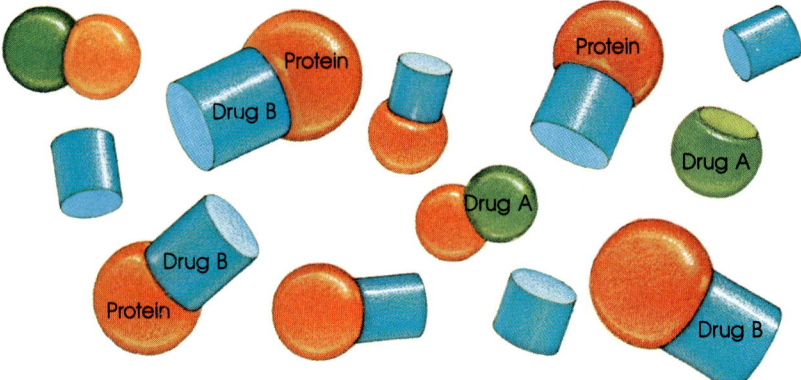

free warfarin is available to bind with receptor sites.

Similar problems arise for patients with conditions, such as chronic liver disease, which reduce albumin concentration. Their free-drug levels rise because fewer proteins than normal are available for binding drug molecules.

The more highly bound a drug is, the more serious the consequences of disturbing its bound/free balance. For instance, freeing an additional 1% of a normally 99%-bound drug like warfarin means doubling the amount of active drug in the system. The body may eventually correct the imbalance by excreting the excess drug. In the meantime, however, the patient could suffer the effects of an overdose.

PROTEIN BINDING: A VARIABLE FACTOR

The extent to which any drug binds to protein depends on the drug's molecular structure. As the examples below demonstrate, binding values vary considerably from one drug to the next.

Warfarin sodium	99%
Diazepam	98%
Furosemide	96%
Dicloxacillin sodium	94%
Propranolol hydrochloride	93%
Tolbutamide	93%
Phenytoin sodium	89%
Quinidine sulfate	80%
Lidocaine hydrochloride	50%
Digoxin	25%

DRUGS AND THE BLOOD-BRAIN BARRIER

Normally, drugs distribute quickly to any area with good blood flow. Yet many drugs never reach the brain, which is one of the most highly vascular organs in the body. Why?

The reason is the *blood-brain barrier:* a protective sheath that restricts the ability of substances in the blood to enter the brain or any other part of the central nervous system (CNS). An endothelium of specialized, tightly joined cells surrounds the CNS capillary walls. This endothelium completely or partially blocks the passage of most water-soluble drugs, though it permits highly lipid-soluble ones to penetrate and take effect quickly. (Water-soluble substances that normally move by active transport—glucose, for instance—penetrate the blood-brain barrier in the same way they do any lipid membrane.) The blood-brain barrier protects the CNS from the toxic effects of many drugs. Penicillin, for example, may cause seizures if it penetrates the brain. Normally, the blood-brain barrier prevents this complication.

Not surprisingly, the barrier complicates the treatment of CNS disorders. When a doctor wants a drug to affect the brain directly, he's limited to using highly lipid-soluble drugs like atropine or sodium thiopental or to injecting the drug directly into the cerebrospinal fluid (CSF). By taking the latter option, the doctor penetrates the blood-brain barrier. The CSF then distributes the drug.

Some CNS disorders (for example, meningitis and encephalitis) impair the blood-brain barrier, permitting drugs to enter the brain. That's why ampicillin and penicillin, which normally don't cross the barrier, can be used to treat meningitis.

UNDERSTANDING DRUG ACTIONS

METABOLISM

LIVER FUNCTION: A REVIEW

The liver, one of the body's most complex organs, is the site of most drug metabolism. Take a moment now to review its anatomy and physiology.

Dark red-brown in color, the liver lies in the upper right part of the abdominal cavity. It weighs more than 3 lb (1.4 kg) in the average man and slightly less than 3 lb in the average woman. Its two lobes contain as many as 100,000 lobules. The 500-plus known tasks the liver performs include:
- secretion of bile (about 1 pint daily)
- metabolism of carbohydrates, proteins, vitamins, fats, and other compounds used by the body
- production of plasma proteins, including enzymes needed for metabolism
- processing of hemoglobin to extract its iron content
- conversion of ammonia to urea
- detoxification of ingested substances (for example, drugs, nicotine and alcohol)
- metabolizes some hormones into inactive (or less active) metabolites
- storage of iron; vitamins A, B_{12}, and D; and glycogen
- synthesis of prothrombin and fibrinogen.

Blood reaches the liver by two separate routes. The hepatic artery brings it oxygen-carrying blood, and the portal vein supplies blood from the digestive tract. Along with nutrients, this blood may contain molecules of an orally administered drug. These molecules undergo first-pass metabolism in the liver. (For more on this process, see the next page.)

Portal circulation

Cross section of a liver lobule
This is the liver's functional unit, where drugs are metabolized.

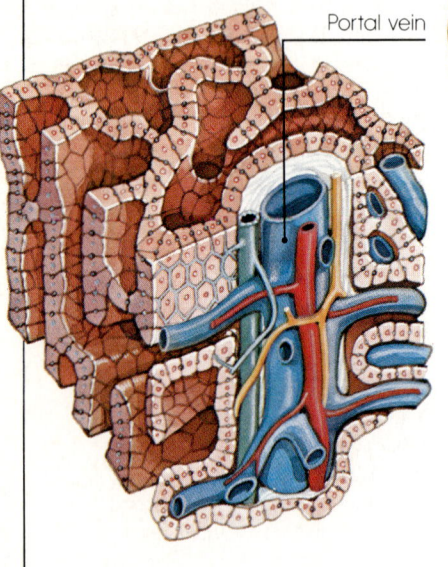

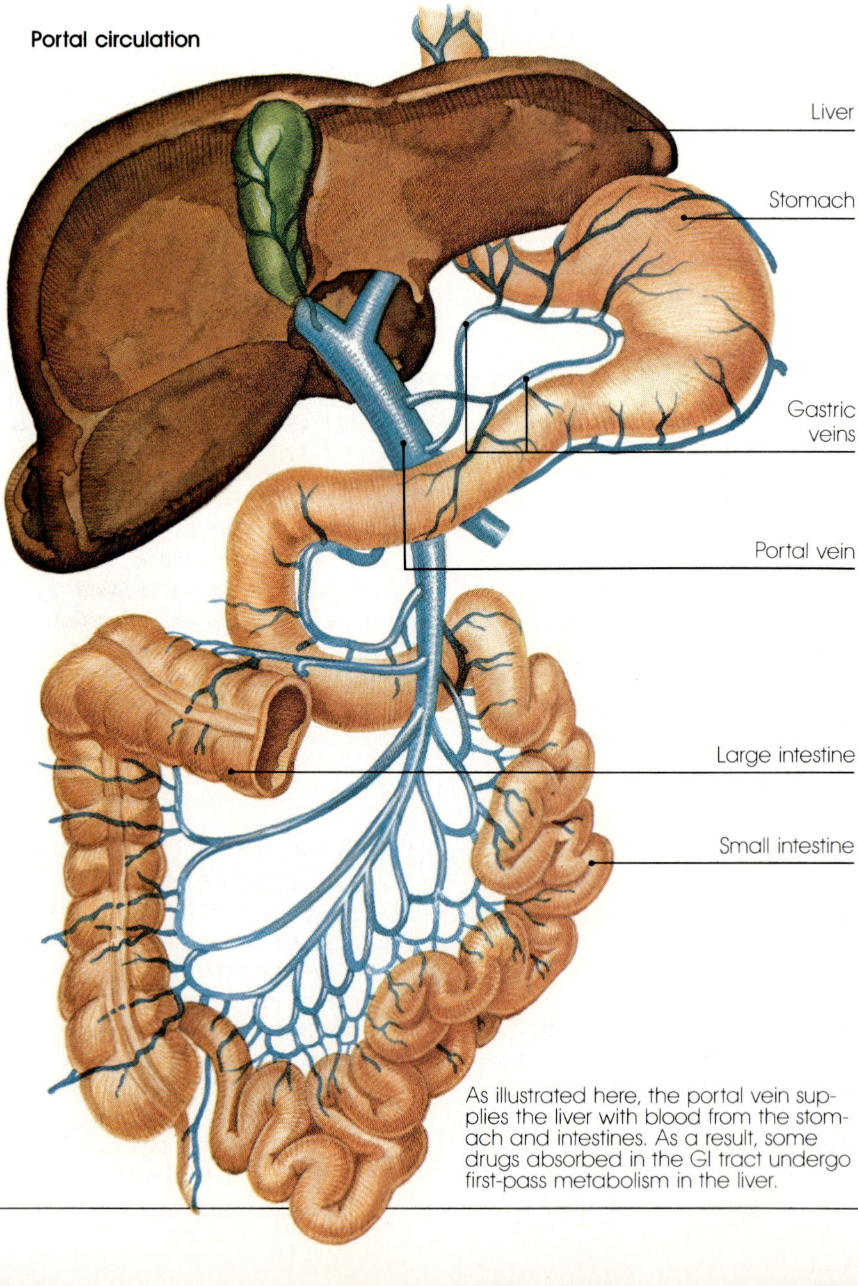

As illustrated here, the portal vein supplies the liver with blood from the stomach and intestines. As a result, some drugs absorbed in the GI tract undergo first-pass metabolism in the liver.

INSIGHTS INTO METABOLISM

How long can a drug continue to affect your patient? At least until it's undergone metabolism, the third step in any drug's progress through the body.

What is metabolism? Metabolism (also called biotransformation) is an interaction between a drug (or other substance) and an enzyme. While the enzyme remains unchanged by the interaction, the drug is broken down into *metabolites* (products of metabolism).

Why is drug metabolism necessary? Because metabolism alters the drug's chemical structure to a more water-soluble form. You'll remember that the more lipid-soluble a drug is, the more easily it crosses cell membranes for absorption into the bloodstream and distribution to receptors. But lipid solubility eases the drug's *inbound* passage only. Water solubility makes the drug easier to excrete.

Where and how. Most metabolism occurs in the liver, which secretes large numbers of the enzymes that *catalyze* the process, or set it in motion. Some metabolism also takes place in the intestinal walls, kidneys, and plasma.

Drug metabolism usually results from action by catalysts called microsomal enzymes. These special enzymes, located mainly in the liver, are nonspecific: they can act on a wide variety of chemical substances. Some drugs (such as phenobarbital) stimulate enzyme activity; others (such as cimetidine) slow enzyme activity.

Pharmacologically active metabolites may be responsible for toxic as well as therapeutic effects.

Four kinds of metabolism. Several different biochemical reactions may take place during the metabolism of a drug from a lipid-soluble to a water-soluble (and hence, excretable) compound.
• *Synthesis* (synthetic reaction): The drug combines with a molecule provided by the body (usually an amino acid or carbohydrate) to form a new substance. This process is also called conjugation.
• *Oxidation:* An oxygen molecule is added to the makeup of the drug compound.
• *Reduction:* An oxygen molecule is removed from the compound.
• *Hydrolysis:* A water molecule is added to the compound, cleaving it.

Metabolites that result from synthesis are pharmacologically *inactive* and ready for excretion. Metabolites resulting from the other three processes are usually pharmacologically *active*. A metabolite formed by any of these last three processes may undergo a subsequent synthetic reaction so that it may be excreted. Some drugs (known as *prodrugs*) are inactive in the form in which they're administered; they don't become active until they're transformed into metabolites.

And for a few drugs, both the administered form and the metabolite are active: codeine and its metabolite morphine, for example.

Patient variables. The rate at which drug metabolism occurs influences both the duration and the intensity of the drug's action. Metabolism rates vary from one person to the next, even among healthy individuals. And a person's normal metabolic rate can be affected by age, genetic disorders, disease (especially of the liver), or drugs in his system.

Because metabolism rates vary so widely among individuals, a standard drug dose may be metabolized into inactivity almost immediately in one patient, yet build up in another's system and cause toxicity. When a patient is taking a medication with a narrow therapeutic index (a narrow range between the minimal therapeutic plasma level and a toxic level), the doctor may order plasma drug studies to help him determine a safe dosage.

A CLOSER LOOK AT FIRST-PASS METABOLISM

As shown on the opposite page, the portal vein brings blood containing nutrients and orally administered drugs from the GI tract directly to the liver. A considerable percentage of these drugs may be metabolized in the liver and sent on to the kidneys for excretion before they ever reach the intended receptor sites.

This process, called *first-pass metabolism*, explains why bioavailability is so much lower for some drugs, such as propranolol, when they're given orally than when they're administered I.V.—and, of course, why oral doses of these drugs must be higher.

Because first-pass metabolism clears some drugs so quickly, oral administration is contraindicated. Oral doses of these drugs would have to be massive to ensure a therapeutic effect. But first-pass metabolism of such massive doses would also produce dangerous levels of active metabolites. Lidocaine is one drug that isn't given orally for this reason.

Note: Some oral drugs are metabolized in the intestine and never reach the liver.

UNDERSTANDING DRUG ACTIONS 25

EXCRETION

UNDERSTANDING EXCRETION
The last step in a drug's passage through the body is excretion. Most drugs go through their final processing in the kidneys and leave the body in urine. (Drugs may also be excreted by the lungs and in feces, saliva, sweat, breast milk, and bile. For more on these excretion routes, see the opposite page.)

The kidneys' role. Excretion by the kidneys involves both the glomeruli and the renal tubules. Excretion occurs by means of active transport and passive diffusion. And the kidneys can excrete both active and inactive metabolites. Let's look at what happens in the process.

• *Glomerular filtration.* In this phase, plasma and its constituents, including molecules of free (unbound) drug, filter through pores in the endothelium of the glomerular capillaries. Macromolecules, such as proteins and protein-bound drugs, remain in the general circulation because they're too large to filter through the pores.

• *Reabsorption.* Passive reabsorption, which takes place in the proximal and distal tubules, is the mechanism for reabsorption of most drug molecules that return from the renal tubules to the bloodstream. Water-soluble drugs are excreted in urine; lipid-soluble drugs are returned to the bloodstream.

• *Active tubular secretion.* Not all drugs can be excreted passively. The renal tubules can excrete some drugs by active transport.

Urine pH: Another factor. You'll remember that ionized drugs are poorly reabsorbed into the bloodstream because they have difficulty diffusing through cell membranes. Urine is normally slightly acidic, allowing weak-acid drugs to remain non-ionized for easy reabsorption into the bloodstream. Weak-base drugs become ionized and therefore aren't reabsorbed. Changing urine pH alters this absorption/excretion relationship. As a result, raising or lowering urine pH may be a valuable therapeutic tool, particularly with drug overdoses. For instance, if a patient has taken too much aspirin (an acidic drug), an alkalizing agent can help his system eliminate the drug faster. If he's taken an overdose of a methamphetamine (a slightly alkaline drug), an acidifying agent ionizes the drug for speedier elimination.

Nursing considerations. Because the kidneys are crucial for the excretion of most drugs, make kidney function assessment a routine part of your nursing care. Follow these guidelines:

• Take a thorough history, asking specifically about past or present kidney problems.

• Monitor laboratory test results, as ordered, especially blood urea nitrogen and serum creatinine values.

• Document fluid intake and output.

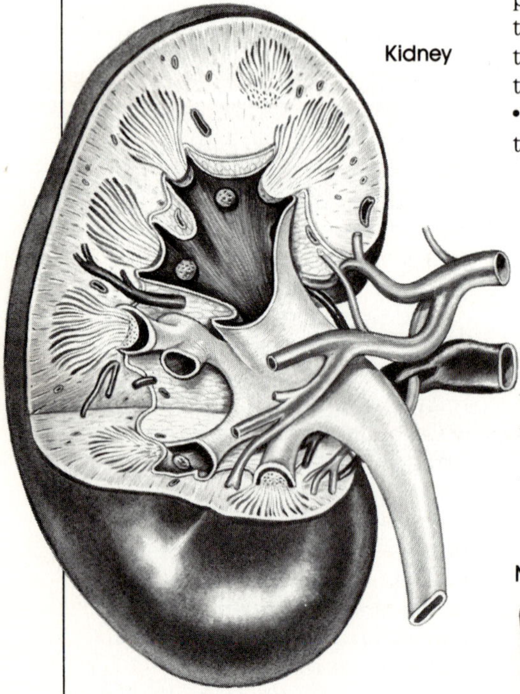

The kidney (shown at left) is the primary site for drug excretion. The nephron illustrated below is the kidney's functional unit, where drugs are secreted into urine or reabsorbed into the bloodstream.

Kidney
- Proximal tubule
- Glomerulus
- Distal tubule
- Collecting duct

Nephron

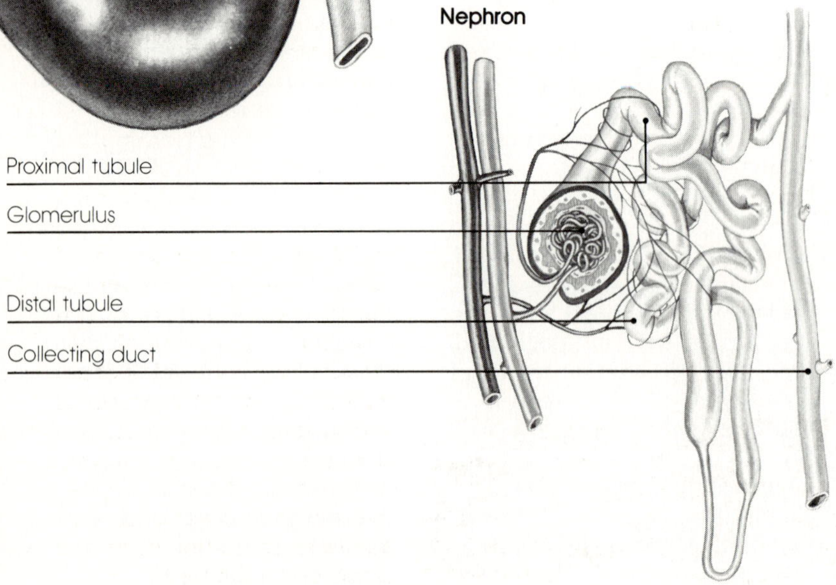

KIDNEY FUNCTIONS—
A QUICK REVIEW

The kidneys lie in the dorsal part of the abdomen, one on either side of the vertebral column. Each kidney is reddish-brown, bean-shaped, and about the length and width of an adult's fist (though not as thick), and contains approximately 1 million nephrons (see page 26 for an example). These structures form a complex filtration network that handles about 200 quarts of blood a day.

The kidneys perform these functions:
• excrete excess water and metabolic waste products
• conserve and reabsorb essential blood substances
• help regulate the plasma's acid-base balance
• regulate plasma volume and electrolyte concentration
• secrete hormones that help regulate arterial pressure, red blood cell production, vitamin D metabolism, and renal blood flow.

Approximately 99% of the fluid that passes through the kidneys is reabsorbed into the circulatory system and sent on through the renal veins. The remainder passes out of the kidneys, through the calices and renal pelvis, to the ureters, bladder, and urethra.

Gallbladder

Common bile duct

The common bile duct carries bile and some metabolized drugs to the small intestine for reabsorption or excretion.

OTHER EXCRETION ROUTES

While the kidneys play the principal role in ridding the body of drugs, a small percentage of drug elimination occurs by other routes. Let's look briefly at each.
• *Bile.* Some drugs and metabolites undergo secretion from the liver into bile and reach the small intestine by way of the common bile duct (see illustration below). From the small intestine, some drugs are reabsorbed into the blood and returned to the liver for metabolism or resecretion into bile. This process, which helps the body retain most of its naturally produced bile acids, is the *enterohepatic* cycle. If the drug is in its active form, the enterohepatic cycle may extend the drug's duration of action far beyond the normal range.

A few drugs secreted into bile continue through the intestines and become part of feces. Excretion by this route is most likely for drugs that are water-soluble; however, lipid-soluble drugs composed of large molecules may also be excreted in feces.
• *Lungs.* The lungs are the main excretion route for anesthetic gases, though small quantities of other drugs may be excreted this way. (In fact, the breathalyzer test given to persons suspected of drunken driving measures alcohol excretion by the lungs.)
• *Intestines.* Unabsorbed drugs that were administered orally may be excreted in feces.
• *Sweat, saliva, and tears.* Small amounts of lipid-soluble drugs may diffuse passively into tear ducts, sweat, and salivary glands and mix with their products. If the patient swallows saliva containing a drug, the drug then takes the same route as any other orally administered substance.
• *Breast milk.* A drug may enter the milk of a lactating woman just as it enters tears, saliva, or sweat—by passive diffusion. Or it may enter by pinocytosis, an active transport mechanism. The chief consequence of excretion by this route, however, involves the suckling infant, since even a tiny concentration of drug may cause problems for him.

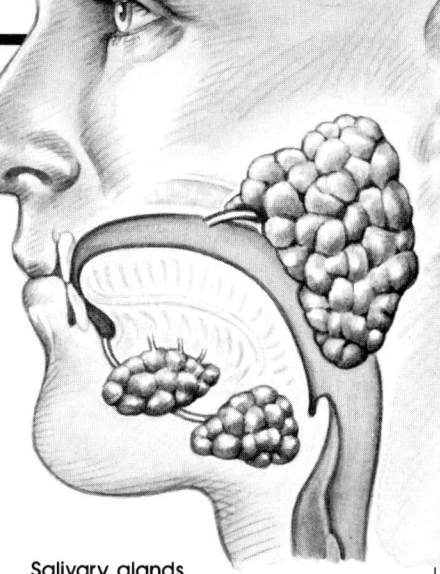

Salivary glands
The three salivary glands (shown above) can secrete small amounts of drugs into the mouth. These drugs may then be swallowed and reabsorbed.

UNDERSTANDING DRUG ACTIONS 27

EXCRETION

DRUG HALF-LIFE AND DOSAGE SCHEDULING

Although drug excretion takes time, many drugs become therapeutically ineffective before excretion is complete. For most (but not all) drugs, the duration of effective action correlates roughly with the drug's *half-life:* the time it takes for its peak (highest) plasma concentration to decrease by half.

Suppose, for example, that a certain I.V. drug has a half-life of 1 hour. This means that 1 hour after administration, the plasma drug level is 50% of the peak level (which is achieved immediately after I.V. administration). At the end of the second hour, concentration is half of the previous level and one quarter of the peak. At the end of the third hour, it's half of the 2-hour level; one eighth of peak.

A drug's half-life may vary from one person to another. This factor is particularly important for the elderly, newborns, and those with physical conditions (such as kidney or liver disease) that alter their ability to handle drugs. For these patients, a drug's usual half-life may be prolonged.

Standard dosage intervals are based on half-life calculations. These figures are helpful in setting up a dosage schedule that builds to a plateau or steady state—a stable drug concentration level that's above the minimum effective level but well below toxicity. *Note:* A steady state can't be achieved for some drugs; for example, penicillin.

DETERMINING A DRUG'S HALF-LIFE

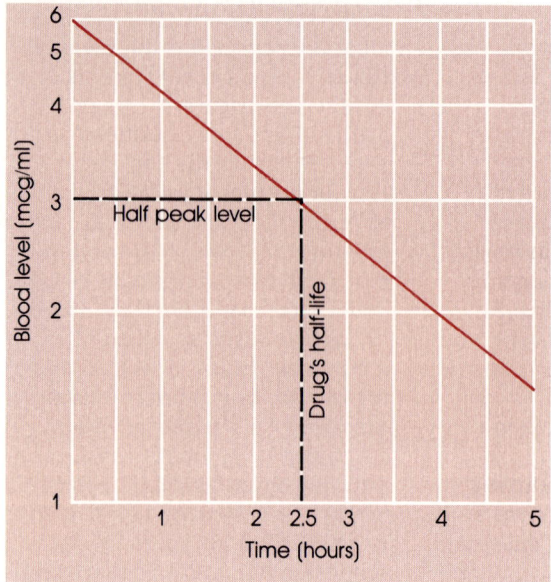

This graph illustrates the half-life of a drug; in this case, gentamicin I.V. As you see, its peak concentration is 6 mcg/ml. Concentration declines to 3 mcg/ml (half of peak concentration) in 2.5 hours; this is the drug's half-life.

REACHING A STEADY STATE

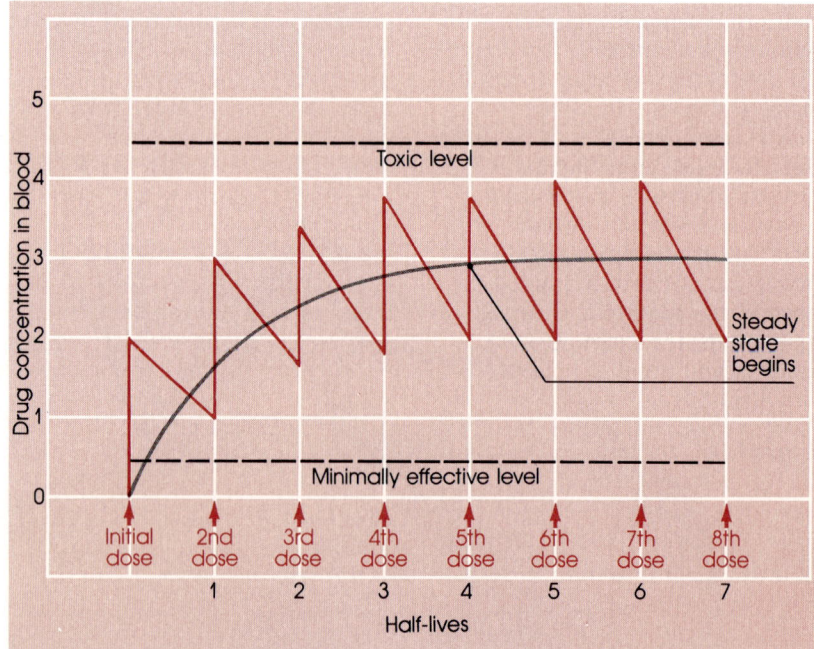

To achieve a therapeutic plateau (steady state) of drug concentration in the blood, the patient receives repeated doses of the prescribed drug at half-life intervals. The drug accumulates so that, after four or five doses on this schedule, the drug amount your patient's receiving equals the amount he's excreting. At this point, plasma drug levels achieve a steady state. As you see in the graph above, the steady state level is safely below the toxic level. *Note:* If therapy begins with a loading dose (for example, when you digitalize a patient), the drug reaches a therapeutic level more quickly.

UNDERSTANDING DRUG ACTIONS

ADVERSE REACTIONS

DRUG REACTIONS: HOW PREVENTABLE?

How many patients experience adverse drug reactions? Too many, say most health-care professionals. Some adverse reactions can't reasonably be anticipated; for instance, an allergic reaction in a patient with no history of allergies. But in most cases, adverse reactions *can* be anticipated—and then, averted or minimized.

Recognizing risks. No drug is entirely free of unwanted effects, and unwanted effects are never entirely predictable. Many factors, including dosage, administration route, and the patient's age and condition, can influence the likelihood of adverse reactions. But these drug types are known to increase a patient's risk:

• drugs with a narrow therapeutic index (see the information at right), including cardiac glycosides, bronchodilators, antineoplastics, antiarrhythmics, and anticonvulsants

• frequently prescribed drugs; for example, analgesics, barbiturates, diuretics, antianxiety agents, antibiotics, and antihypertensives

• highly potent drugs, especially those which tend to interact with other drugs; for example, anticoagulants and corticosteroids.

Patient history. Along with knowing the drug's characteristics, knowing your patient and his health history is a vital part of preventing drug interactions. (See page 8 for a review of critical questions to ask him.) If he tells you that he's had problems taking any drugs or other substances, find out exactly what the problems were and document them. Be particularly careful when questioning geriatric patients, who are likely to be taking several medications, including over-the-counter ones.

ADVERSE REACTION OR SIDE EFFECT?

When a drug produces an unintended response, is the response an adverse reaction or a side effect? Both terms have defenders—and some authorities use both, reserving the term *side effect* for an unwanted but predictable drug effect and *adverse reaction* for a serious or unpredictable result.

But the term you and your patients will encounter consistently in package inserts and other literature from the Food and Drug Administration (FDA) is *adverse reaction*, which the FDA defines as:

> "...an undesirable effect, reasonably associated with the use of the drug, that may occur as part of the pharmacological action of the drug or may be unpredictable in its occurrence."

This definition covers allergies and toxic reactions as well as intensifications of normal activity. Throughout this book, you'll see the term *adverse reaction* used for any unintended and undesirable response to drug use.

WEIGHING RISKS AND BENEFITS

When will a doctor choose to prescribe a drug he knows can produce serious adverse reactions? He'll consider several questions before making the decision:

How wide is the drug's therapeutic index? Therapeutic index (the range between minimally effective and toxic plasma drug levels) determines a drug's margin for dosage error. If a drug's therapeutic index is wide, the patient can safely tolerate plasma drug levels well above the minimally effective level; as a result, adverse reactions are less likely. But if a drug's therapeutic index is narrow, the margin for error is small. Therefore, maintaining drug levels within the safety range is more difficult and the risk of adverse reactions is higher.

How serious is the patient's condition? The answer to this question helps the doctor decide if a drug's benefits outweigh its risks for the patient. If the patient is suffering from an uncomplicated respiratory infection, the doctor won't order a high-risk anti-infective, such as chloramphenicol, which may cause fatal aplastic anemia.

If the patient has a life-threatening salmonella infection, however, this drug may offer the best chance for recovery.

A narrow therapeutic index is particularly significant if the drug is likely to accumulate in the patient's system; for example, because he's elderly or has a kidney condition.

How dangerous is the adverse reaction? The mouth dryness that cholinergic blockers commonly produce is bothersome but not life-threatening. Compared with the drug's benefits, this adverse reaction is acceptable. But oral contraceptives, which may cause thrombophlebitis in susceptible women, are an unacceptable birth-control option for patients at high risk of this adverse reaction—especially since other birth-control options are available.

How easily can the patient adjust to the adverse reaction?

CONTINUED ON PAGE 30

UNDERSTANDING DRUG ACTIONS

ADVERSE REACTIONS

WEIGHING RISKS AND BENEFITS CONTINUED

Some adverse reactions are minor inconveniences that can be minimized: by taking prazosin at bedtime, for instance, the patient can avoid first-dose orthostatic hypotension. Other drug reactions, such as drowsiness from methyldopa, may disappear after a week or so of treatment. But some reactions are so unpleasant, severe, or prolonged that they discourage your patient from taking his medication.

Take special care to teach your patient about the adverse reactions he may experience: how to minimize or avoid them, if possible, and how to cope with them, if necessary. For example, if constipation is a common adverse reaction, suggest dietary changes to minimize this problem.

In addition, keep these guidelines in mind:
• Tell the patient to inform the doctor about *any* reactions he experiences—even if they seem insignificant or if they're not reactions he's been taught to expect.
• Teach him how to recognize allergic and other adverse reactions. Have him notify his doctor at once if he experiences any serious adverse reaction.
• Encourage him to consult his doctor or pharmacist before treating any reaction with over-the-counter (OTC) drugs. Emphasize that OTC drugs may mask serious adverse reactions—or cause additional problems by interacting with the prescribed drug.
• Help him plan a diet that's compatible with his drug regimen. If he's taking a drug whose action is affected by diet (for example, an anticoagulant), encourage him to maintain a consistent diet.
• Discuss the importance of taking his drugs as prescribed, and tell him what to do if he misses a dose.
• Explain how alcohol can prolong drug effects. If appropriate for the drug he's taking, instruct him to avoid alcohol.
• Urge him to undergo periodic laboratory evaluations, if appropriate, to ensure effective therapy and reduce the risk of adverse reactions.

ADVERSE REACTIONS: SOME POSSIBLE CAUSES

What causes an adverse reaction? In many cases, you may not be able to identify a single cause. The patient's condition or his unique response to a particular drug can play an important part. But in many cases, the problem can be traced to the drug itself—its dosage, administration route or rate, or formulation. For details about each factor, read on.

Inappropriate dosage. An excessive drug dose generally results in the intensification of the drug's normal pharmacologic effects. An excessive dose of an anticoagulant is more likely to cause hemorrhaging; similarly, an overdose of diuretics can cause serious depletion of electrolytes and body fluid.

Although some overdoses are accidental, others result from *overcompliance;* for example, the patient may decide that two doses of a drug are better than one. If an asthmatic patient tries to relieve his breathing difficulties by overusing his bronchodilator, the drug may become ineffective and his condition will worsen.

Route and rate changes. Varying a drug's administration route or rate can enhance or diminish its effect. Oral administration results in slower and usually lower bioavailability, so a switch from oral to I.V. or I.M. administration without a dosage change may intensify drug response. Too-rapid I.V. infusions may also trigger unexpected adverse reactions; for example, hypocalcemic tetany from tetracycline infusion and cardiac dysrhythmias from lincomycin. Frequency can also be a problem: psoriasis patients taking frequent small doses of methotrexate are more likely to develop cirrhosis and fibrosis than those taking intermittent large doses.

Formulation problems. A change in product makeup can make a difference, too. Formulation changes that result in a more highly purified product can intensify the patient's response. For example, highly purified insulin given in the same dosage as a less-pure formulation may cause hypoglycemia. Similarly, removing inert substances from a product can increase bioavailability and produce a functional overdose, as has happened with some preparations of phenytoin, digoxin, and tolbutamide.

Formulation factors affect liquid medications, too. In a poorly prepared liquid medication, the active ingredient may form a highly concentrated sediment. A liquid-only dose of this medication would have almost no therapeutic value, while one with a large amount of sediment could contain a dangerously high amount of drug. And, of course, any drug that's past its expiration date may no longer act as intended and could even cause toxicity.

CRITICAL QUESTIONS

IDENTIFYING ADVERSE REACTIONS

Spotting an adverse reaction isn't always easy. The signs and symptoms, time of onset, and degree of severity vary widely from one drug to another and from patient to patient. But if you know your patient and the characteristics of the drugs he's taking, you can minimize problems. If your patient is taking a drug that you know produces adverse reactions, ask him if he's experiencing any of those reactions. For instance, long-term administration of procainamide hydrochloride (Pronestyl) may produce drug-induced lupus erythematosus syndrome. If your patient has been taking procainamide for over 6 months, ask him if he's experiencing any aches or pains in his fingers. He may not think to report these minor arthralgias, but they're consistent with early signs of lupus.

If you suspect that your patient is having an adverse reaction, investigate further by asking yourself these questions:

- When did the change in his condition occur—before, during, or after drug therapy? (Remember, adverse reactions can be delayed for several weeks.)
- Is this symptom related to his condition or disease?
- What's the ordered dosage? Is the dosage schedule within the normal range for the drug, given the patient's condition and age?
- Is the patient allergic to other drugs?
- Has he ever had this symptom when taking another drug that's similar to the drug he's taking now?
- Does he have any condition, such as a liver or kidney disorder, that could be a contributing factor?
- Have you noted any changes in his laboratory values or urine output?

If you determine that he's experiencing an adverse reaction, ask yourself:

- Is the reaction an enhancement of normal drug response (in other words, is it dose-related)?
- Is the doctor likely to reduce the drug dosage, or will he discontinue the drug entirely?
- Does the patient need additional treatment?
- Is he taking any other drugs (for example, an OTC drug) that could be contributing to the reaction?

DRUG TOXICITY: PREDICTABLE AND PREVENTABLE

Drug toxicity results when too much drug accumulates in a patient's system. Any factor that tends to encourage drug accumulation or to slow metabolism or excretion—for example, excessive drug dosage or impaired renal or liver function—may lead to toxicity.

Toxicity can cause several effects: an *intensification of the desired pharmacologic effect* (such as barbiturate overdose, causing excessive central nervous system depression), a *worsening of adverse reactions* associated with the drug (for instance, hemorrhage from an anticoagulant), or a combination of the two. Most drug toxicity is predictable and dose-related; most can be reversed by adjusting dosage.

Toxicity types. Drug toxicity is categorized as follows:

- *Acute toxicity* occurs within a short time, following administration of one (or several) excessive doses. It can be accidental or deliberate. (Suicide attempts fall within this category.)
- *Chronic toxicity* results from drug buildup over time because more drug has entered the circulatory system through absorption than has left it through metabolism and excretion. A patient with impaired renal function who's also taking digoxin may not experience digoxin toxicity for several weeks after drug therapy begins. During this time, the drug gradually accumulates to toxic levels because the kidneys can't excrete the drug fast enough.

Those patients receiving a phenothiazine drug, such as chlorpromazine hydrochloride (Thorazine, Largactil) for the long-term treatment of psychosis, are at high risk of chronic drug

CONTINUED ON PAGE 32

UNDERSTANDING DRUG ACTIONS

ADVERSE REACTIONS

DRUG TOXICITY: PREDICTABLE AND PREVENTABLE CONTINUED

toxicity. Possible signs and symptoms include tremors, rigidity, shuffling gait, and other parkinson-like symptoms; difficulty swallowing or breathing; and extreme motor restlessness.

Your role. To protect your patient from drug toxicity, focus on prevention and early detection. Follow these guidelines:
• Take a thorough history. Identify problems, such as a kidney or liver condition, that predispose the patient to toxicity.
• If the doctor prescribes a nephrotoxic drug, ask him to order kidney function studies before and during therapy. (Check hospital policy; serum creatinine and blood urea nitrogen studies may be routine for patients taking certain nephrotoxic drugs, such as tobramycin.)
• If the patient's taking a drug that may affect his vision or hearing, perform a gross visual acuity or hearing acuity assessment. Continue assessment throughout therapy.

Drugs with a narrow therapeutic index, such as digoxin, may cause toxicity even if plasma drug values remain at normally nontoxic levels. That's why you must closely monitor your patient for signs and symptoms of toxicity.

• During therapy, document your patient's fluid intake and output, observing especially for signs of kidney dysfunction (such as oliguria). Inform the doctor of changes in urine output.
• Monitor the patient for physiologic changes (especially kidney and liver problems). Keep a watchful eye on plasma drug level results and other laboratory values, if ordered. Inform the doctor of significant changes.
• Teach the patient to maintain the dosage schedule set up by the doctor. Stress the importance of taking his drugs exactly as ordered.
• Teach him to recognize the signs of toxic buildup for the drug he's taking and the steps to take if toxicity develops.
• Stress to your patient the importance of obtaining routine laboratory tests after discharge to check plasma drug levels or other laboratory values as ordered by the doctor.

BUILDING A DRUG TOLERANCE

A patient who's repeatedly given a particular drug may develop a *tolerance* for it. In other words, his response to the original dose decreases to the point that he needs larger doses to achieve the desired effect.

Tolerance results from a change in the drug's rate of passage through the body, an increase in microsomal enzyme activity (which speeds drug metabolism), or a reduction in reactivity at receptor sites. Humans aren't the only organisms that become tolerant of drugs, of course. Bacteria exposed to repeated low concentrations of an antibiotic gradually become resistant to it.

Tachyphylaxis, or acute tolerance, occurs when a patient develops tolerance in a short period of time; the bronchodilator ephedrine sulfate can set off this reaction, as can morphine sulfate in large doses. Cross-tolerance is also common: many individuals who have developed tolerance to one drug in a group become unresponsive to other related drugs.

Tolerance and toxicity. With higher tolerance for a drug, does an individual's toxic threshold for the drug rise? That depends.

Tolerance is a particular risk with drugs that affect the central nervous system, such as stimulants, barbiturates, and narcotics.

Someone with a tolerance for morphine, for instance, may show no ill effects from doses well above normal limits. On the other hand, toxic doses of alcohol and barbiturates are just as dangerous for habitual users of the drugs as they are for abstainers.

When a patient stops taking a drug, his tolerance for it disappears—slowly with some drugs, rapidly with others. If your patient has become drug-tolerant, the doctor must choose between changing treatment entirely and increasing dosage to an effective level. His decision depends on the effects of the drug itself, the expected duration of treatment, and the possibility of finding another drug that's not closely related to the drug the patient's developed a tolerance for.

32   UNDERSTANDING DRUG ACTIONS

ALLERGY

A QUICK REVIEW

Without question, an allergic drug reaction is one of the most serious adverse reactions your patient can experience. What provokes such a reaction? Although no one knows all the answers, a review of the normal immune response provides some clues. Take a moment to consider what follows.

As you'll recall, an antigen is any substance that provokes an immune response. Normally, the body produces antibodies (also called immunoglobulins) to combat specific antigens that threaten well-being. Antibodies bind to mast cells throughout the body and to basophils circulating in the blood. Then, when an antibody encounters its corresponding antigen, it binds with it to form a macromolecule called an antigen-antibody (Ag-Ab) complex. The Ag-Ab complex causes the mast cell or basophil to break apart and release vasoactive substances, including histamine, which help destroy the antigen. This process, called the *immune response*, is the body's way of protecting itself from harmful invaders.

In an allergy, however, the body mistakenly recognizes a benign substance as a threat. The resulting antigen-antibody reaction causes the symptoms of allergy, which vary in quality and intensity according to the allergy type and the patient's individual response. In short, the immune system goes awry, causing an abnormal and possibly dangerous overreaction.

THE MAKING OF A DRUG ALLERGY

An almost limitless number of usually benign substances, including drugs, can trigger allergic reactions in susceptible individuals. A drug allergy occurs when the drug provokes antibody formation, as we've just discussed, causing an adverse reaction that's unrelated to the drug's pharmacologic action. Now, let's examine drug allergy in more detail.

Stage I: Forming antibodies. When an allergy-producing drug first enters the body of a susceptible individual, it's unlikely to cause any symptoms. Nevertheless, it's starting to cause trouble. For reasons not fully understood, the body recognizes the drug as an antigen and begins making antibodies. This process takes from several days to more than a week. Most likely, the drug has been eliminated from the patient's system by then, which explains why the patient doesn't experience an allergic reaction on first exposure to the drug. But when he's again exposed to the offending drug, he's almost certain to experience an allergic reaction of some sort.

Stage II: Allergic reaction. As in a normal immune response, an allergic response triggers release of histamine and other vasoactive substances from mast cells and basophils. But because an allergic response is abnormal and excessive, this process causes adverse reactions that can range from a rash or hives to anaphylactic shock. These reactions may appear within seconds (following an I.V. injection, for example) or days later.

Allergic response to a drug can vary from one individual to the next: penicillin may give one person a mild rash and another anaphylactic shock, with no apparent reason for the difference.

Even the same patient may

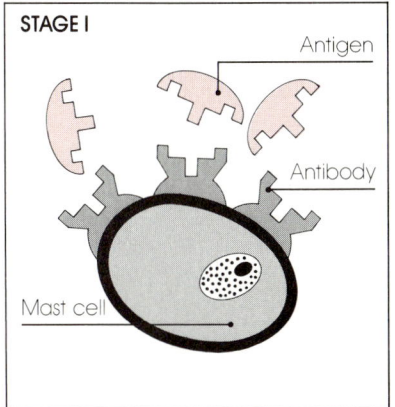

In response to an antigen, antibodies begin forming on a mast cell.

During an allergic reaction, antigens and antibodies combine, as shown here, breaking up the mast cell and releasing vasoactive substances.

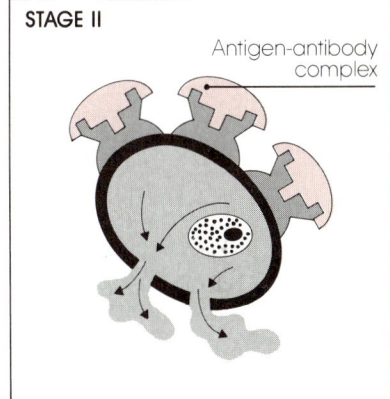

react differently at different times. Once an allergy has appeared, however, the individual is likely to experience an allergic response of some sort every time he encounters the drug itself or others with similar structure.

Because no one can be sure an individual *isn't* allergic to a given drug, the doctor may reserve drugs that frequently provoke an allergic response—penicillin, for instance—for use when no comparably effective alternative exists.

Serum sickness. By the time antibodies are ready to circulate, the antigens that provoked them

CONTINUED ON PAGE 34

UNDERSTANDING DRUG ACTIONS 33

ALLERGY

THE MAKING OF A DRUG ALLERGY CONTINUED

have usually left the body. But if some antigen remains in the circulatory system, antigens and antibodies can form complexes that circulate, lodge in small blood vessels, and produce *serum sickness*—a less acute systemic allergic reaction that appears 1 to 3 weeks after drug administration. Skin rashes, joint swelling, stiffness, and fever are the characteristic symptoms—though liver, kidney, and bone marrow damage may also result.

Long-acting procaine penicillin frequently sets off this illness; streptomycin, sulfonamides, and thiouracils have also been linked to it. In most cases serum sickness is no worse than uncomfortable, and symptoms disappear within a week. But bronchospasm and other more complicated reactions may also appear with the disorder, and symptoms can linger as long as 6 weeks.

Drug route considerations. How a drug enters the body seems to influence its risk for provoking an allergic reaction. Topical administration is apparently the most likely to sensitize a patient for future reactions; oral administration the least likely.

With penicillin, the oral route provokes far fewer allergic reactions than do parenteral routes—roughly half as many. More than 100 deaths from anaphylaxis after parenteral administration are reported every year, but only a few occur in patients receiving penicillin orally.

TOPICAL DRUGS: HANDLE WITH CARE

Because topically applied drugs have great potential for provoking sensitivity reactions, protect both yourself and your patient by taking the following precautions.
• Wear gloves when applying topical drugs, to protect yourself from a sensitivity reaction. If you don't wear gloves, take care to thoroughly wash your hands after the procedure.
• Scrupulously follow administration directions. Applying an excessive drug dose increases your patient's risk of developing a sensitivity to the drug.
• Before applying a transdermal drug, thoroughly cleanse the previous drug dose from the site. Apply the new dose onto clean, dry, unbroken skin.

Important: Wash your hands after preparing injectable drugs. The drug preparation procedure may cause aerosolizing, permitting skin contact with airborne drug droplets.

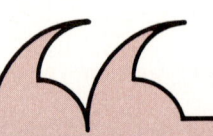

"Although you can't always predict drug hypersensitivity, your patient's history can warn you of potential problems. Is he allergic to seafood, eggs, or other foods? Does he suffer from hay fever or any other environmental allergy—for example, to feathers, mold, or dander? If so, he may be prone to drug hypersensitivity."

Yuki Yumibe, RN, MSN
Associate Professor in Nursing
Pacific Lutheran University
Tacoma, Washington

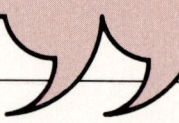

IS YOUR PATIENT REALLY ALLERGIC?

You're performing an admission assessment for Mrs. Burton, who has just been admitted with a diagnosis of cholecystitis. When you ask her about allergies, she tells you, "I'm allergic to codeine."

Note her response—but don't stop there. Ask her what her symptoms were, why codeine was prescribed, and whether she discussed the problem with her doctor. You may learn that the codeine she was given for pain relief after an appendectomy 12 years ago upset her stomach. Because no one warned her that codeine often causes GI distress, she assumed that she had an allergy.

Mrs. Burton is one of many patients who mistake a fairly minor adverse reaction for an allergy—and in doing so deprive themselves of a large class of drugs.

Other patients have misconceptions about what an allergy is. For example, your patient may claim to be allergic to penicillin. On investigation, however, you may find that some other family member is allergic to penicillin and that your patient in fact has never received it. He's just assumed that the allergy is hereditary.

Your careful questioning and follow-up teaching can reopen the door to better treatment for him. Follow these guidelines:
• Explain the difference between an allergic reaction and other adverse reactions.
• Teach him how to avoid or minimize adverse reactions.
• Encourage him to discuss any adverse reactions he experiences with his doctor. By adjusting dosage or substituting another drug, the doctor may be able to minimize the problem.

UNDERSTANDING DRUG ACTIONS

ANAPHYLAXIS

IDIOSYNCRASY: AN UNPREDICTABLE DANGER

You know the standard safeguards against hypersensitivity reactions: taking a careful drug history and withholding a drug if your patient has a history of allergic reaction to it (or a related drug or substance). But these measures are useless for preventing an unusual but serious hypersensitivity reaction called *idiosyncrasy*. Unlike an allergic reaction, idiosyncrasy doesn't result from antigen-antibody formation following first exposure to a drug. Instead, it apparently stems from a genetically determined intolerance of a particular drug. A patient may develop an idiosyncratic reaction without warning, on first exposure to only a small amount of a drug.

Known idiosyncratic reactions range from mild to severe and may include the following: photosensitivity, alopecia (secondary to dry scalp), purpura, rashes, exfoliative dermatitis, systemic lupus erythematosus, blood dyscrasias (including aplastic anemia, hemolytic anemia, agranulocytosis, and thrombocytopenia), hepatotoxicity, malignant hyperpyrexia, nervous system damage (including extreme muscle weakness), ototoxicity, and nephrotoxicity.

A few of these reactions disappear when the drug is stopped, but others cause permanent damage. Your responsibility is to be aware of the drugs known to provoke idiosyncratic reactions; for example, tetracyclines, phenothiazines, ampicillin, phenytoin, chloramphenicol, phenylbutazone, methimazole, valproic acid, furosemide, and ethacrynic acid. Use such drugs with caution, observe the patient carefully for adverse reactions, and teach him to recognize and report signs and symptoms.

RECOGNIZING ANAPHYLACTIC SHOCK

Anaphylactic shock, a life-threatening, systemic allergic response, is one of the most alarming experiences imaginable, for your patient and you. Learn about it—including how to recognize it *immediately*—by reading what follows; then, we'll discuss how to intervene.

Anaphylactic shock occurs when an antigen—such as a drug, a food or food-derived dye, snake or insect venom, or an antigen present in a blood transfusion—reacts with an antibody to trigger a generalized, severe allergic reaction. The vasoactive substances released cause smooth-muscle contraction, especially in lungs, leading to bronchospasm. They also cause increased vascular permeability and vasodilation. As shown below, these effects lower blood pressure and lead to shock. Respiratory distress develops rapidly; death can follow within minutes.

By quickly spotting the condition, you give your patient the best chance of survival. Immediately suspect anaphylaxis if he's experiencing chest tightness (a classic symptom), respiratory distress (dyspnea, wheezing, choking, cyanosis), itching, urticaria, erythema, or angioedema. Check him for GI complaints and signs of vascular collapse: rapidly falling blood pressure, thready pulse, sweating, weakness, anxiety, and dizziness. Call for help—and be ready to start the countermeasures described on the following page.

How anaphylaxis develops

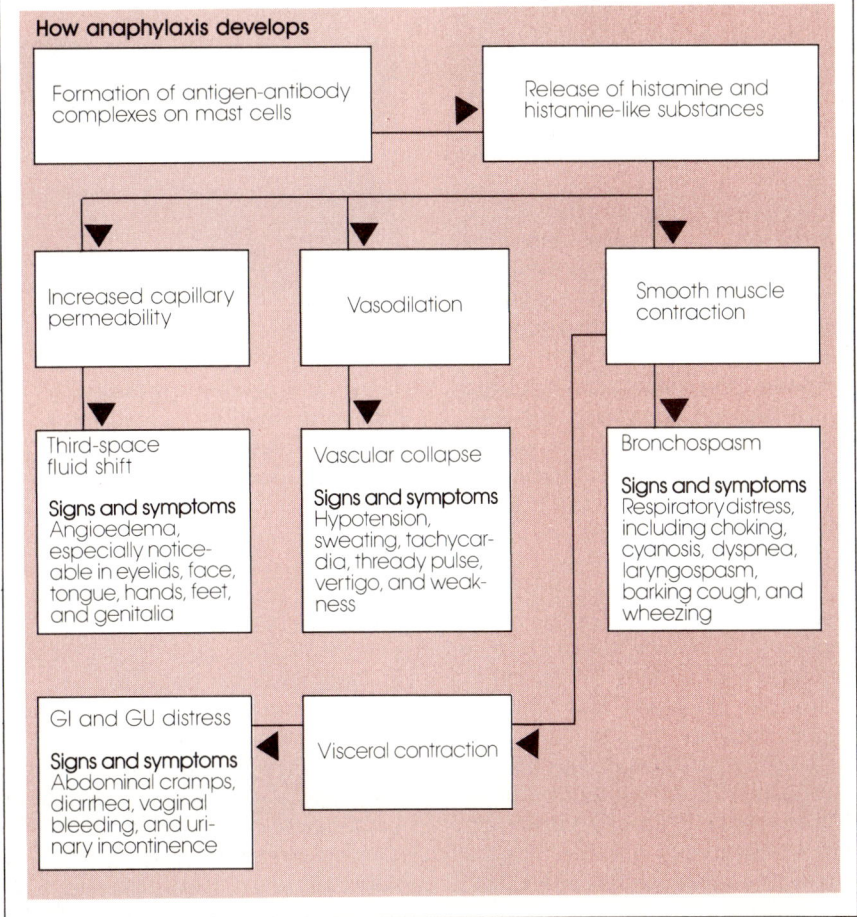

Formation of antigen-antibody complexes on mast cells → Release of histamine and histamine-like substances

→ **Increased capillary permeability** → **Third-space fluid shift**
Signs and symptoms: Angioedema, especially noticeable in eyelids, face, tongue, hands, feet, and genitalia

→ **Vasodilation** → **Vascular collapse**
Signs and symptoms: Hypotension, sweating, tachycardia, thready pulse, vertigo, and weakness

→ **Smooth muscle contraction** → **Bronchospasm**
Signs and symptoms: Respiratory distress, including choking, cyanosis, dyspnea, laryngospasm, barking cough, and wheezing

→ **Visceral contraction** → **GI and GU distress**
Signs and symptoms: Abdominal cramps, diarrhea, vaginal bleeding, and urinary incontinence

UNDERSTANDING DRUG ACTIONS

ANAPHYLAXIS

How to intervene

A flashing light at the nurses' station alerts you to check on Ms. Collins, a 27-year-old lawyer who was admitted yesterday for drainage of an abscess. As you enter the room, you notice that she's flushed and sweaty. She tells you that her chest feels tight and she's hot, itchy, and dizzy. Auscultating her lungs, you hear wheezing; you also observe swelling in her hands and face.

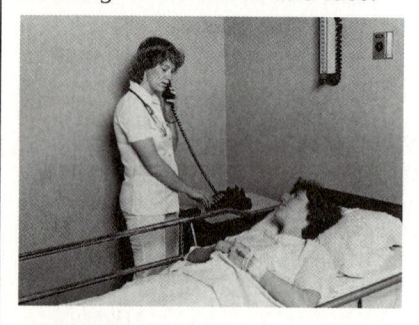

You immediately recognize the most likely cause of Ms. Collins' symptoms: anaphylaxis. What should you do? Call for help—stat. Then, take the steps detailed below.

Important: Never leave your patient to go for help. Remember, anaphylactic shock can be fatal within minutes. Until help arrives, you may be your patient's only chance.

• *Keep the patient's airway open and provide respiratory support.* Release of histamine and similar substances increases capillary permeability and causes fluid shift (angioedema). Assess airway patency and be prepared to intubate the patient if laryngeal edema sets in. (The doctor may decide to perform an emergency tracheotomy.) Also, be prepared to insert an airway and perform CPR, if necessary.

• *Look for obvious causes.* If your patient is receiving medication intravenously, stop the drip—or, if she has only one I.V. line, slow it to a keep-vein-open rate. You may need the line shortly to administer drugs and fluids. Insert a second I.V. line as soon as possible.

If your patient's alert, ask her if she's had any medication or eaten any food in the last hour.

Important: Don't waste precious seconds looking for a cause. If nothing is immediately obvious, go straight into emergency treatment.

• *Check your patient's vital signs.* Look particularly for evidence of hypotension. If her blood pressure is dropping, lay her flat or raise her feet to encourage venous return to the heart. A thready pulse is further confirmation of anaphylactic shock.

• *Administer oxygen.* Give oxygen at a low-flow rate, unless the doctor directs otherwise.

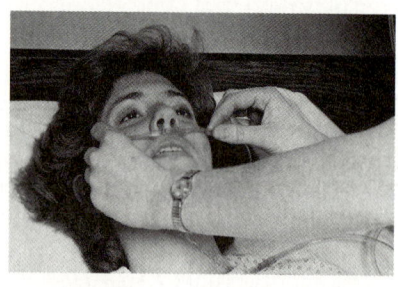

• *Administer appropriate medication.* Release of vasoactive substances, including histamine, causes edema, bronchospasms, and vasodilation, which lowers blood pressure. Epinephrine hydrochloride (Adrenalin) and diphenhydramine hydrochloride (Benadryl) are both histamine antagonists; the doctor will probably order both drugs.

Epinephrine, administered first, actively reverses the effect of histamine and raises blood pressure by causing vasoconstriction. It also eases bronchospasms and the visceral contractions that can cause GI and genitourinary discomfort. As ordered, give epinephrine in a 1:1,000 dilution: 0.3 to 0.5 ml subcutaneously, 1 ml intramuscularly (I.M.), or an I.V. bolus of 0.1 to 0.25 ml. As needed, repeat at 10-minute intervals.

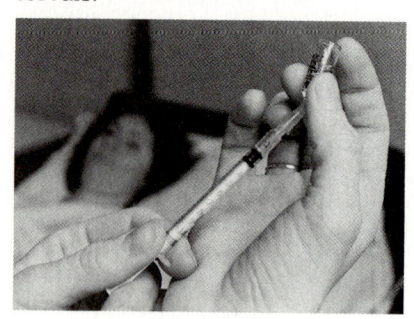

Addition of the antihistamine Benadryl (50 to 100 mg I.V., I.M., or orally) blocks histamine from reaching additional receptor sites. Epinephrine and Benadryl together may be all the treatment your patient requires.

• *Reassure your patient and provide ongoing support.* She's anxious—understandably, under the circumstances; anxiety is characteristic of anaphylactic shock. Let her know that you're staying with her and that help is on the way.

Also, remember that reversing the vasoconstriction associated with shock may be painful. So continue to support and reassure your patient during recovery.

• *Administer fluids.* If your patient's shock symptoms haven't disappeared after medication administration, the doctor may order an I.V. infusion of normal saline solution or Ringer's lactate solution to help restore normal blood pressure.

• *Administer additional drugs, as needed.* The doctor may order a vasopressor like norepinephrine (Levophed) by I.V. infusion: 4 mg (1 amp) in 500 ml of I.V. solution run at 8 to 12 mcg/minute at first, then 2 to 4 mcg/minute.

If the patient's attack was severe, the doctor may also order a

36 UNDERSTANDING DRUG ACTIONS

corticosteroid, such as dexamethasone (Decadron), to prevent further systemic reaction. To relieve continuing bronchospasms, he

Don't forget that an unconscious patient can still hear. Take care with what you say during resuscitation efforts.

may also order aminophylline. Give a loading dose of 6 mg/kg over at least 30 minutes; then 0.3 to 0.7 mg/kg/hour continuous infusion or intermittent bolus. For oral administration, give 500 mg initially, then 250 to 500 mg every 6 to 8 hours.

• *Document treatment.* On your patient's chart, document what happened, including the patient's signs and symptoms, all medical and nursing interventions, and the outcome of treatment.

• *Monitor your patient.* Continue watching your patient closely, even after her vital signs have stabilized. Watch for adverse reactions to the emergency treatment she's undergone as well as for signs of recurring shock.

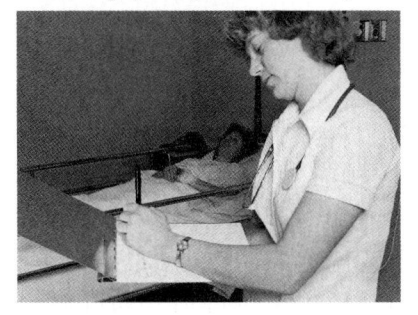

Note on her chart that she shouldn't receive any vasodilators for the next 24 hours, since this may cause her blood pressure to drop again. If she's going home, warn her not to take any drugs without her doctor's approval or to drink alcoholic beverages; explain that a hot bath or shower could also cause problems.

Important: If the allergy-causing drug was a sustained-release preparation, symptoms may recur. Monitor the patient closely. If she's leaving the hospital, stress the importance of taking the antihistamines the doctor prescribes, exactly as directed.

• *Think ahead.* If you haven't already identified the allergen that caused your patient's anaphylaxis, help her to trace back and find the problem. (Keep in mind that anaphylactic shock develops within an hour of contact with the antigen.) *Important:* Some patients have been known to receive 16 courses of penicillin treatment with no complications, yet go into anaphylactic shock on the 17th. Don't exclude any drug as a possible cause of the reaction just because your patient has tolerated it before.

When you've identified the cause, note your findings on your patient's chart, warn her to avoid the substance in the future, and explain the importance of wearing a Medic Alert tag. Make sure she understands that she must let all other health-care professionals who deal with her know about the problem. Document the allergy and the reaction on her records in red.

Caution: Your patient may be equally sensitive to other drugs with similar molecular structure: penicillin-allergic patients often can't take a cephalosporin for this reason. And, in general, patients who have developed an allergy to one substance are more likely to develop allergies to others. Know your patient's history. If he's reported an itchy rash from certain foods or animals, he's more likely to develop drug allergies as well.

WHEN NO OTHER DRUG WILL DO

The range of drugs available is so wide that a doctor can almost always find an effective substitute for an allergy-causing drug. Occasionally, though, the offending drug is the only one that can help the patient. In such cases, a doctor—usually an allergist—may perform a desensitizing procedure. A patient being desensitized receives small but gradually increasing doses of the drug he's allergic to over a few hours, until he's taking a standard dose.

If you're caring for a patient undergoing this procedure, watch him carefully for signs of allergic reaction, so that emergency intervention can begin the moment trouble develops. If your patient's an outpatient, continue to observe him for 30 minutes after drug administration. Make sure you know emergency protocol for the area you're working in. (With a drug like penicillin, which provokes life-threatening reactions in some patients, the procedure takes place in an intensive care unit or other facility equipped to deal with emergencies.)

After desensitization is complete, take care to give the patient his medication on schedule. (If he's an outpatient, emphasize the importance of following his prescription exactly.) Also, make sure he understands that desensitization isn't a cure—his hypersensitivity will return after the current course of drug therapy ends.

NURSING CONSIDERATIONS

Drug administration: considering the options

What's the best way to give a drug? That depends, of course, on the answers to a variety of questions. Is the patient's condition acute or chronic? Life-threatening or just a nuisance? Is he hospitalized or caring for himself at home? Does he have any physical, emotional, or economic problems that may affect compliance or increase the risk of adverse drug reactions?

The doctor considers these and many other questions whenever he decides on a drug, route, and dosage. But you play an important role, too. As part of your nursing assessment, you know details about the patient's history and life-style that may affect compliance and the effectiveness of therapy. As a result, you can alert the doctor to potential problems and influence his choice of drug type and route.

For example, suppose your patient is a traveling salesman with an unpredictable schedule. For convenience, he may prefer a sustained-release capsule (if his medication is available in that form) or a drug that has a long half-life and can be taken only once a day. Similarly, an elderly patient who has difficulty swallowing tablets may prefer a liquid medication. By making drug administration as convenient as possible for the patient, you encourage his compliance.

For background on the various drug forms and administration routes available, read the following pages carefully.

Comparing drug routes

A drug's administration route influences absorption and distribution, which, in turn, affect drug action and patient response. Which administration route is best for your patient? Consider the following points.

TOPICAL

Advantages
- Easily administered
- Provides fast relief for itching and topical pain
- Isn't likely to cause severe allergic reactions (unlike systemic routes)
- Causes fewer adverse reactions than systemic routes
- Some drugs (for example, nitroglycerin and scopolamine) may be applied topically (in a form called transdermal skin patches) for prolonged systemic effects.

Disadvantages
- Dosage accuracy may be difficult to achieve.
- May stain clothing or bedding
- Drugs applied for systemic effect may cause unexpected adverse reactions if administered carelessly. For example, scopolamine applied as an antiemetic may cause more pupil dilation than usual if the drug is accidentally transferred to the eyes from the fingertips.
- Drugs applied for topical effect may be absorbed systemically, causing problems.

ORAL

Advantages
- Allows for easy self-medication
- Economical
- Drug retrieval or dilution possible with lavage or vomiting in cases of overdose

Disadvantages
- Unsuitable for most emergencies because of relatively slow absorption rate
- Unpredictable absorption, which may limit drug reliability
- May be metabolized during first pass through the liver
- May irritate the GI tract, discolor the teeth, or have an unpleasant taste
- May be accidentally aspirated if patient has difficulty swallowing or is combative
- Unsuitable for self-medication if the patient isn't capable of managing his own therapy. Oral drugs are also potentially dangerous in households where small children may ingest them.

SUBLINGUAL OR BUCCAL

Advantages
- Permits drug to take effect quickly, since it's absorbed directly into the bloodstream
- Can be used if patient can't swallow, if he's intubated, or if he can't take anything by mouth for any other reason
- Avoids first-pass effect in the liver
- Prevents GI tract irritation

Disadvantages
- May be used only for drugs that are highly lipid-soluble
- Not useful if drug has an unpleasant taste
- Can irritate oral mucosa

RECTAL

Advantages
- Provides a safe route if the patient is vomiting, unconscious, or unable to swallow for any other reason
- Provides an effective route to treat vomiting
- Doesn't irritate the patient's upper GI tract, as some oral medications do
- Protects medication from destruction by digestive enzymes in the stomach and small intestine

Disadvantages
- May be uncomfortable and embarrassing for the patient
- Is usually contraindicated when the patient has a disorder affecting the lower GI tract; for example, rectal bleeding or diarrhea
- May result in irregular or incomplete drug absorption, depending

38 UNDERSTANDING DRUG ACTIONS

on the patient's ability to retain the medication and whether feces are present in his rectum. Because rectal absorption may be incomplete, rectal doses of some medications may be larger than oral doses.
• Unsuitable for most emergencies because absorption is unreliable.
• May irritate rectal mucosa
• May stimulate the patient's vagus nerve by stretching his anal sphincters. For this reason, use the rectal route cautiously with cardiac patients.

RESPIRATORY
Advantages
• Provides rapid drug absorption and distribution because of the lungs' large surface area and rich capillary network
• Allows for smaller doses of potent drugs, minimizing their systemic adverse reactions
• Easily accessible, providing a convenient alternative when other routes are unavailable. In emergencies, some injectable drugs (such as epinephrine) can be given directly into the lungs, where they're quickly absorbed.
• Useful for administering drugs that are both lipid-soluble and available as gases
Disadvantages
• Dosage accuracy may be difficult to achieve.
• Some drugs may cause nausea and vomiting.
• May cause tracheal or bronchial irritation, resulting in coughing or bronchospasm
• May lead to hand-held nebulizer dependency (for example, in an asthmatic patient)
• The full drug dose may be difficult to administer by hand-held nebulizer; for example, if the patient is an uncooperative child. *Note:* Hand-held nebulizers are a potential infection source.
• Relatively few drugs can be given by this route.

PARENTERAL
All parenteral routes are potentially useful for treating a patient who can't receive medication by the oral route; for example, because he's unconscious. And all of them avoid the risk of decreased drug absorption from vomiting or gastric activity. Listed here are some specific advantages and disadvantages for each parenteral route.

INTRAVENOUS
Advantages
• Drug is immediately bioavailable, making this route the first choice for emergency drug administration and for immediate or long-term pain relief.
• Absorption into the bloodstream is complete and reliable.
• Provides a route for some medications, such as dopamine hydrochloride (Intropin), that can't be given by any other route
• Enables delivery of large drug doses at a continuous rate
• Avoids causing muscle tissue damage from potentially irritating drugs
• Avoids first-pass effect in the liver
Disadvantages
• May cause life-threatening adverse reactions if administered too rapidly, if I.V. flow rate isn't carefully monitored, or if incompatible drugs are mixed. (Mixing incompatible drugs may also cause precipitation, lessening the drug's effectiveness.)
• Increases risk of complications, such as extravasation, vein irritation, systemic infection, or air embolism

INTRAMUSCULAR
Advantages
• Allows administration of aqueous suspension, solutions in oil, or medications that aren't available in oral form
• Ensures long-term absorption of suspensions or solutions in oil, by forming a medication deposit
• Allows administration of parenteral medications in relatively large doses (up to 5 ml)
• Eliminates the need for an I.V. site
• Achieves a relatively rapid effect
Disadvantages
• Medication may precipitate in the muscle, reducing absorption.
• Medication may not be properly absorbed if the patient is hypotensive or has poor blood supply to the muscle for any other reason.
• Injection may damage blood vessels, causing bleeding.
• Medication may be accidentally injected into the bloodstream, possibly causing overdose or an adverse reaction.
• Injection may damage nerves, causing unnecessary pain or paralysis.
• Injection may damage bone.
• Injection may cause pain and local tissue irritation.
• By damaging muscle tissue, injection may interfere with cardiac isoenzyme reading ordered to help diagnose myocardial infarction.

SUBCUTANEOUS
Advantages
• Permits easy self-administration of insulin for diabetic patients
• Permits a drug, such as insulin, to be absorbed slowly, prolonging the drug's effects
• Provides rapid absorption while avoiding the need for an I.V. site
Disadvantages
• May damage skin tissue
• May not be used when patient has occlusive vascular disease with poor perfusion, since decreased peripheral circulation delays absorption
• May not be used when patient's skin tissue is grossly adipose, edematous, burned, hardened, swollen at all the common sites, damaged by previous injections, or diseased

NURSING CONSIDERATIONS

UNDERSTANDING BIOAVAILABILITY

The doctor may select a drug form on the basis of its *bioavailability*, or the extent to which the drug is absorbed. Generally, a change in drug form or administration route that enhances bioavailability also enhances the patient's response to drug therapy.

Complete bioavailability is achieved almost immediately via the I.V. route. All other routes provide slower and less predictable absorption patterns.

Absorption by the oral route is particularly unpredictable for several reasons. In addition to the effects of the GI tract, an oral drug's bioavailability is influenced by the pharmacochemical properties of a capsule or tablet (such as rate of disintegration and dissolution in the GI tract), amount and type of inert ingredients (including preservatives), the patient's age and physical condition, and numerous other factors.

ORAL DRUG TYPES: SPECIAL CONSIDERATIONS

Because oral drugs are prescribed so frequently, you may be inclined to take their administration for granted. After all, swallowing a pill isn't complicated for most patients. But keep in mind that oral drugs (tablets, capsules, and liquids) must be handled like any other drug type—knowledgeably and carefully, to ensure effective and safe treatment.

Read the following information for a review of the special considerations appropriate for each oral drug type. As you'll see, each has unique features that affect how you administer it—and what you teach your patient.

CAPSULE
Powdered, granulated, or liquid drug encased in a gelatin shell; solid drug particles may be coated for sustained-release action

- Because the gelatin shell dissolves quickly in the GI tract, the drug is readily available for absorption. As a result, a drug in capsule form may take effect more quickly than a drug in tablet form.
- Be alert for signs of deterioration, such as discoloration and unusual odor. Check the expiration date.
- Instruct the patient not to chew capsules.

TABLET
- Teach the patient how to properly divide a scored tablet, if ordered. But don't divide a tablet that isn't scored.
- Never crush enteric-coated tablets.
- Don't give enteric-coated tablets with milk or antacids. Doing so raises the stomach's pH level, causing the tablets to dissolve prematurely.
- Don't crush sustained-release tablets.

SYRUP
Drug in a viscous, sugar/water solution; usually flavored

- When giving a syrup for a soothing effect, tell the patient to sip it slowly. For best results, don't follow it with water.
- You may dilute most syrups given for systemic effect. But dilute only the dose you're giving. In addition to affecting the dosage, dilution can destroy the syrup's preservative and hasten contamination or decomposition.
- As with any drug, check the expiration date. Also, examine the solution for cloudiness or precipitation; depending on the drug, these conditions may indicate a loss of effectiveness.
- Use caution with a diabetic patient. If he's a *brittle* diabetic, check with the pharmacist to see if a sugar-free syrup is available.
- When giving syrups with other drugs, administer syrups last.
- Remind the patient to store syrups (and all drugs) out of children's reach.

SUSPENSION
Drug suspended in water; for example, magmas, gels, and emulsions

- Thoroughly shake a suspension before giving it.
- If desired, you may dilute most suspensions with water before administration.

ELIXIR
Mixture of drug, alcohol, water, and sugar

- Check the solution for precipitate. If the mixture has precipitated, don't administer it.
- If the ordered dose is over 4 ml, double-check the order; elixirs are usually ordered in small doses.
- To dilute the solution, use only a small amount of water. Too much

UNDERSTANDING DRUG ACTIONS

water could cause the drug to precipitate.
- Consult the pharmacist before you mix elixirs with liquids other than water.
- Follow the elixir with water (unless the drug is ordered for cough relief, since water may reduce the elixir's soothing effect).
- Store the solution in an airtight container and protect it from temperature extremes.
- Use caution if your patient is alcoholic. *Caution:* Never give an elixir to a patient receiving disulfiram (Antabuse).

RECONSTITUTED POWDERS AND TABLETS

Powdered drugs or tablets reconstituted with water or other liquid

- Read the directions carefully before reconstituting powders and tablets. Don't use too much water with effervescent tablets or they'll boil out of the glass.
- Allow effervescent tablets to dissolve completely.
- Give the drug without further dilution.
- Some powders (for example, potassium chloride) become gelatinous very quickly after mixing. Mix them at the patient's bedside and administer them immediately.

SPECIAL NOTE: Some drugs may be administered in solution. If they're acidic solutions, such as diluted hydrochloric acid, they can damage tooth enamel. Administer such drugs with a glass straw.

HOW FOOD AFFECTS DRUGS

Before you administer an oral drug, always check when—and what—the patient ate last. Although in some cases food in the stomach has little effect, it can retard or prevent absorption of some drugs. Yet with other drugs, food enhances absorption. Knowing how food affects the drug you're giving may enable you to ensure proper absorption and avoid adverse reactions, such as nausea, dyspepsia, and diarrhea.

Drugs administered orally undergo several changes before entering the patient's systemic circulation. For example, a tablet disintegrates and dissolves before being absorbed through the intestinal mucosa. Stomach pH affects the rate and degree of dissolution. So, when food changes stomach pH, the drug absorption rate and degree may also change.

Food stimulates several body secretions, most importantly gastric acid and bile. For this reason, you'll give some drugs when the patient's stomach is empty, so gastric secretions won't adversely affect absorption. But you'll give fat-soluble drugs *with* meals, because bile helps dissolve them.

Keep in mind that food delays stomach emptying. So a drug given with meals may remain in the stomach longer, delaying the therapeutic effect. To ensure a more rapid effect, administer the drug when the patient's stomach is empty.

By acting as a buffer, food also minimizes GI distress, nausea, and mucosal damage resulting from ulcerogenic drugs, such as aspirin and indomethacin (Indocin*).

*Not available in Canada

WHAT'S IN A TABLET?

A tablet (or capsule) contains more substances than the drug itself. In fact, the drug may make up a relatively small portion.

This pie graph illustrates the proportions of substances that may be contained in one penicillin potassium tablet.

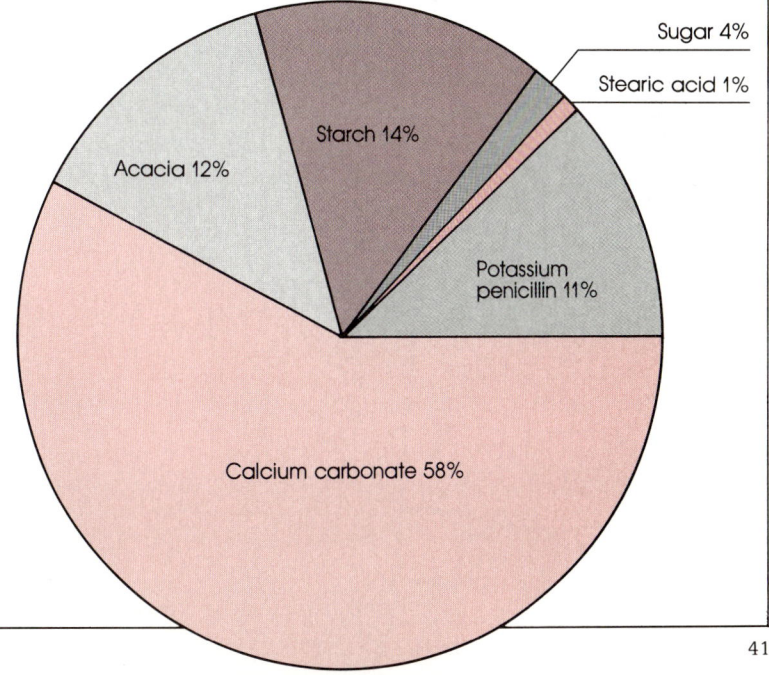

- Sugar 4%
- Stearic acid 1%
- Starch 14%
- Acacia 12%
- Potassium penicillin 11%
- Calcium carbonate 58%

NURSING CONSIDERATIONS

WHAT YOU SHOULD KNOW ABOUT CRUSHING TABLETS

What if your patient has difficulty swallowing his medication? You may want to crush a tablet or open a capsule to make administration easier. But, to make sure you can *safely* do so, read the following guidelines.

Generally, you may crush tablets and open capsules. (Some capsules—for example, those containing pediatric doses—are specially designed to be opened.) Then you can mix the medication with a beverage or a small amount of soft food, such as applesauce or mashed potatoes, before administering it. But, before mixing any medication with a food or beverage, be sure to check that the drug's action won't be affected. And since the medication may alter the food's taste, tell your patient what you've done.

But never crush a sustained-release or enteric-coated tablet. Remember, the special coating is designed to ensure proper absorption at the right time, in the right place. If you crush a sustained-release tablet, the entire dose is available for absorption all at once, instead of over a period of hours. A drug overdose could result. Similarly, crushing an enteric-coated tablet destroys the drug's protective coating. As a result, the drug will dissolve in the stomach instead of the small intestine, possibly causing gastric irritation or even vomiting.

You may open a sustained-release *capsule* and mix its contents with food or water. But take care to mix the drug *gently*, not vigorously.

Note: Check with the pharmacist before crushing any tablets. He may be able to provide a liquid form of the drug or prepare a special formulation. But, if he says you can safely crush the tablet, be sure to clean the mortar and pestle before you begin and after you're through. (Or, if you're using other equipment, such as a cup, make sure it's clean.) Doing so prevents drug errors due to particles left on the equipment.

Now, examine the information below for more details.

Drug manufacturers may use these designations to indicate the sustained-release drug form:

Dura-Tabs
Extentabs
Gradumets
Gyrocaps
Repetabs
Sequels
Spansules
Tembids

When attached to a drug name, these words and abbreviations indicate the sustained-release form.

Bid
CR
Dur
LA
Plateau Cap
SA
Span
SR

Don't crush enteric-coated and sustained-release tablets or vigorously mix sustained-release capsules.
Here are some examples:

Aminodur Dura-Tabs*
Artane Sequels
Azulfidine EN-tabs*

Bayer Timed-Release Aspirin*

Chlor-Trimeton Repetabs*
Combid Spansules
Compazine Spansules*

Desoxyn Gradumets*
Diamox Sequels*
Dimetane Extentabs
Dimetapp Extentabs*
Donnatal Extentabs
Drixoral
Dulcolax

Ecotrin
Elixophyllin SR
E-Mycin

Feosol Spansules*

Indocin SR*
Isordil Tembids

K-Tab*
Kaon-Cl*
Klotrix*

Modane

Nicobid*
Nitro-Bid Plateau Caps*
Nitrospan*

Ornade Spansules*

Pavabid Plateau Caps*
Peritrate SA
Peritrate with Phenobarbital SA
Polaramine Repetabs
Procan SR*

Quibron-T/SR*
Quinaglute Dura-Tabs
Quinidex Extentabs*

Slo-Phyllin Gyrocaps*
Slow-K

Tedral SA
Theo-Dur*
Theolair-SR
Theophyl-SR
Thorazine Spansules*
Trilafon Repetabs

Valrelease*

Because of a peculiarity in their makeup, these drugs shouldn't be mixed or crushed.

Azo-Mandelamine*

Depakote*
Doraphyl*

Ery-Tab*
Eskalith CR*

Inderal LA

Mandelamine
Micro K Extencaps

Nitrostat SR
Norpace CR

Povan Filmseals*
Pronestyl-SR*
Pyridium

Ritalin SR*

Theoclear L.A.*

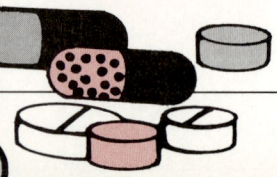

Zorprin*

*Not available in Canada

GENERICS

GENERIC DRUGS: A SAFE SUBSTITUTE?

As patients become better informed about health care, they're bound to have more questions about drug therapy. And one of the questions you're most likely to hear is "Can the doctor prescribe a generic drug for me?"

Although you can answer *yes* in most cases, you should be aware of some important exceptions. Read what follows for general guidelines.

Generic versus brand names. A generic drug name is the chemical description of the drug; a brand name (or trade name) is the name chosen by a drug company for marketing purposes. For example, *phenytoin sodium* is a generic name; *Dilantin* is a brand name.

Although generic drugs are usually less expensive than their brand-name counterparts, using them can cause problems—especially if they're used interchangeably with a brand-name counterpart during a course of therapy. Why? Surprisingly, generic and brand-name drugs are *not* always bioequivalent, even though they contain the same amount of the same drug. The reason could be differences in nondrug ingredients; for example, diluents or disintegrants. Or the drugs may be subject to different manufacturing processes. These and other factors can cause drugs to become bioavailable at different rates.

Although some experts disagree, most generic drugs are roughly bioequivalent with their brand-name counterparts and substitutions can be made safely. But some drugs shouldn't be substituted after a course of therapy begins. This is especially important for drugs with a narrow therapeutic range, such as digoxin and levothyroxine.

Your role. By all means, encourage your patient to ask his doctor or pharmacist about generic drug use, especially if he's undergoing long-term therapy. And, if possible, suggest to the doctor that he *begin* therapy by ordering a generic drug, to avoid the problems that a later substitution may cause. By prescribing a generic drug, the doctor may save the patient a substantial amount of money.

If the doctor prescribes a generic drug, give the patient this advice:

• Instruct him to check with the pharmacist (or doctor) if the pharmacist refills the prescription with a drug that's a different color than the one your patient is accustomed to. The pharmacist may have substituted one generic drug for another. If so, he and the doctor must make sure that the new generic drug will affect your patient in the same way as the one he took previously.

• Tell him to inform the doctor if the generic drug doesn't seem to be as effective as the brand-name drug—or if he notices any effects that the previous drug didn't cause.

"I have mixed feelings about substituting a generic drug for a brand-name drug after a course of therapy has begun—especially if therapeutic dosage was difficult to establish for the patient. While the generic drug may be more economical for the patient, it also introduces an element of uncertainty to the treatment. Remember, the patient may not respond in the same way to the generic drug. If he was responding well to therapy with the brand-name drug, why upset the applecart?"

Larry N. Gever, RPh, PharmD
Springhouse, Pa.

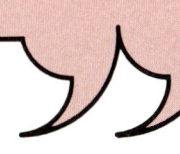

"For a great many drugs, substituting one brand for another is quite safe. Hydrochlorothiazide is a good example. The various generic and brand-name versions of this drug are essentially bioequivalent; substituting one for another has no appreciable effect on therapy. If substitution saves the patient some money without affecting therapeutic response, then I'm all for it."

J. Ken Walters, BS, PharmD
Hartford Hospital
Hartford, Connecticut

UNDERSTANDING DRUG ACTIONS

LEARNING ABOUT DRUG INTERACTIONS

How often do drug interactions occur? Probably more frequently than you think, because drug interactions are easily mistaken for adverse drug reactions. But the distinction is important, because you must identify the problem correctly before you can intervene appropriately.

Drugs simultaneously present in the body have opportunities to interact at each stage of drug processing: absorption, distribution, metabolism, and excretion. Or they can interact at receptor sites. If the action of one or more drugs changes as a result, your patient could experience an unwanted—and potentially dangerous—drug interaction.

But not all interactions are dangerous. In fact, if you think that drug interactions are harmful by definition, you'll be surprised to learn that some can actually be exploited for the patient's benefit. The interaction between penicillin and probenecid, for example, can help a patient by prolonging penicillin's action in the body.

For details on these and other points, as well as practical information on how to minimize your patient's risks, read on.

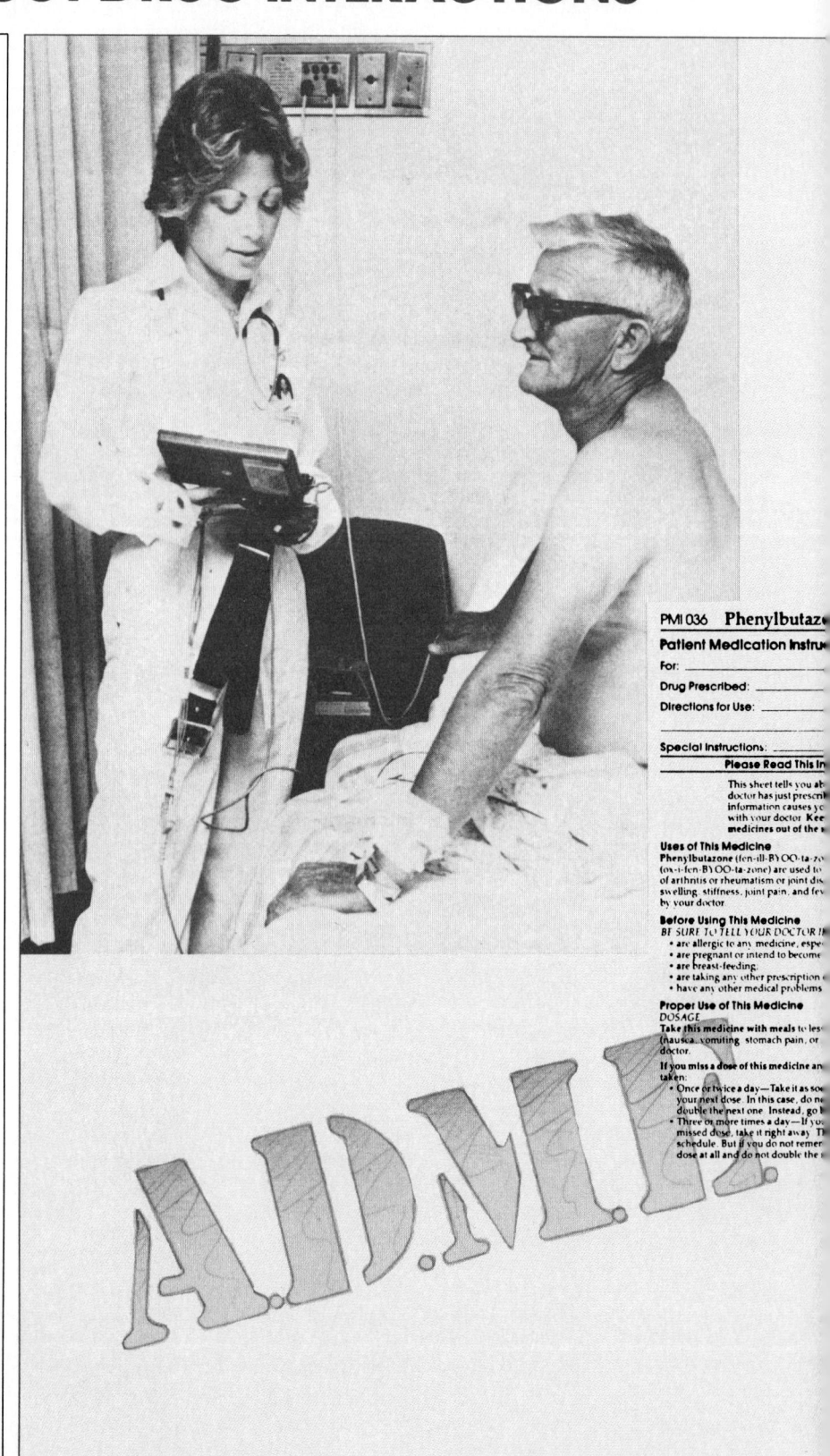

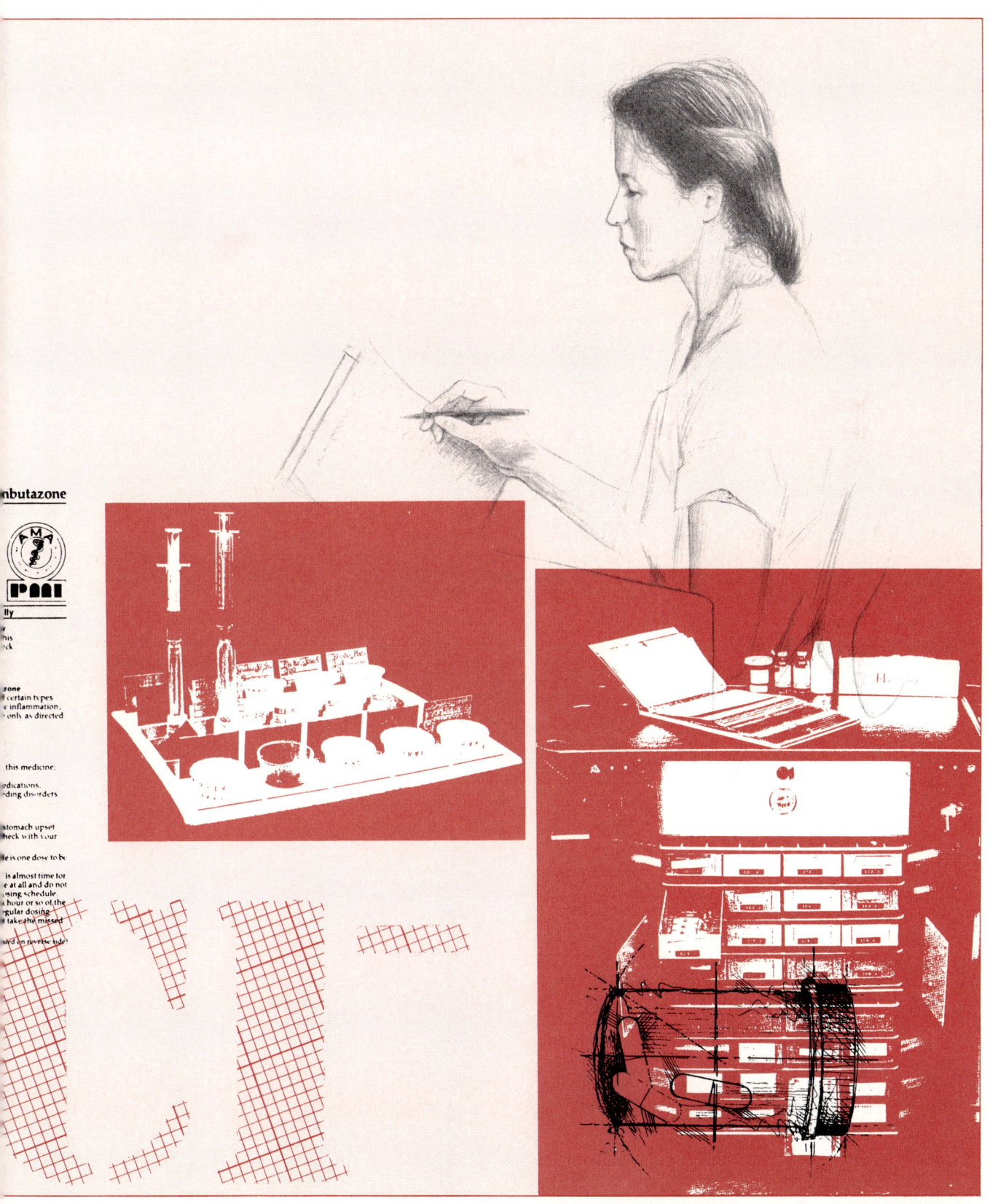

LEARNING ABOUT DRUG INTERACTIONS 45

GENERAL CONCEPTS

DRUG INTERACTIONS: SEEING BOTH SIDES

Although some drug interactions cause adverse reactions, others can be exploited for the patient's benefit. Consider the following case histories to see how these drug interactions had three different outcomes.

Case history #1. Myra Walton, a 69-year-old retired librarian, suffered a myocardial infarction 6 months ago. To treat the mild congestive heart failure that developed during recovery, the doctor prescribed digoxin 0.25 mg P.O. and furosemide (Lasix) 40 mg P.O. daily.

Because Mrs. Walton recently began having chest pains, her doctor admitted her for observation. As part of her admission workup, he ordered a plasma digoxin level, which revealed a therapeutic concentration of 1.8 ng/ml. He continued digoxin therapy at the same dosage.

Mrs. Walton's baseline EKG showed that she was experiencing paroxysmal atrial tachycardia (PAT). To control the PAT, the doctor ordered verapamil 80 mg P.O. t.i.d. Then, he sent her to the ICU for continuous cardiac monitoring.

A few days later, Mrs. Walton began to experience nausea and loss of appetite. Within a few more days, she began vomiting, developed frequent premature ventricular contractions, and complained of green-tinted vision. That morning's plasma digoxin level revealed an alarmingly high level: 3.2 ng/ml. Even though Mrs. Walton's digoxin dosage didn't increase during her hospitalization, she showed a level consistent with digoxin toxicity. Why?

The reason is an interaction between digoxin and verapamil. Verapamil causes plasma digoxin levels to rise by an average of 70%, according to one recent study. The two drugs *can* be given together safely—but only if the patient's digoxin dosage is lowered by 40% to 50% and plasma digoxin levels are closely monitored.

Fortunately, Mrs. Walton suffered no long-term ill effects. The doctor immediately stopped her digoxin and finally, one week later, her digoxin values returned to a therapeutic level. Then, the doctor resumed digoxin therapy, but at half the previous dosage: 0.125 mg daily.

Case history #2. Edward Kinney, age 52, is admitted to your hospital with chest pains and shortness of breath. Diagnostic tests reveal a pulmonary embolism. While taking his history, you learn that Mr. Kinney is a diabetic and that he controls his condition with tolbutamide (Orinase).

Initially, Mr. Kinney's placed in the ICU and started on heparin I.V. Then, once his condition stabilizes, his doctor switches him to dicumarol P.O. and has him transferred to your unit.

You watch closely for bleeding and monitor his prothrombin time (PT) daily. When Mr. Kinney's PT increases, you hold the dicumarol for 1 day, as ordered. Then, laboratory studies reveal a blood sugar drop. As ordered, you hold the tolbutamide for a day, as well. Mr. Kinney's blood values then return to baseline.

Why did Mr. Kinney experience these adverse reactions? While taking both tolbutamide and dicumarol, he was the victim of a *double drug interaction*. In other words, the drugs interact mutually, changing each drug's normal effects. Dicumarol inhibits the metabolism of orally administered tolbutamide, potentiating its hypoglycemic effect. Simultaneously, tolbutamide displaces dicumarol from protein-binding sites, increasing the anticoagulant effect.

Case history #3. Now, consider the example of Victor Simmons, who comes to your clinic complaining of pain during urination and a penile discharge. The diagnosis is gonorrhea. As ordered, you give probenecid 1 g P.O. Then, you give him 4.8 million units of aqueous procaine penicillin G, I.M., divided and administered at two different sites.

You know that penicillin is the drug of choice for gonorrhea. But why does the doctor order probenecid? In this case, he's using a drug interaction to the patient's advantage. Normally, penicillin is rapidly excreted from the body, so its beneficial action lasts only a short time. But probenecid inhibits the active secretion of penicillin at the kidneys' proximal and distal tubules. As a result, plasma and tissue levels of penicillin remain high for a longer period, and the drug's action is prolonged.

HOW TO CLASSIFY DRUG INTERACTIONS

As the case histories above illustrate, a drug interaction can be adverse or beneficial. Regardless of the result, when most drugs interact their effects can be classified in one of these categories:
• pharmacokinetic—one drug's effects may alter the absorption, distribution, metabolism, or excretion of another drug.
• pharmacodynamic—the drugs' effects may be additive (the total effect of two drugs together equals the sum of their individual effects), synergistic (the combined effect is greater than the sum of their individual effects), or antagonistic (one drug blocks all or part of another's effect).

ASSESSING YOUR PATIENT'S RISK

Is your patient at risk of drug interactions? The number of drugs he's taking, along with his age and physical condition, can help you assess the potential for problems. Consider these points.

High-risk patients. Any patient who takes several drugs a day is at special risk of drug interactions. *Polypharmacy*—the concurrent administration of several drugs—is a common feature of medical treatment today. Because medicine has become so highly specialized, a patient may be under the care of several doctors. And he may receive prescriptions from each. Interactions may subsequently occur because one doctor doesn't know what another has prescribed. Add to this any OTC drugs the patient uses, and the risk increases.

As the number of drugs a patient uses increases, so do the risks of noncompliance, dosage or timing errors, and other examples of drug misuse. These factors make interactions more likely.

The elderly, who generally take two to three times more drugs than do younger adults, are at risk for this reason. But they're also at risk because the aging process tends to reduce kidney and liver function, which affects drug metabolism and excretion.

Young patients are at risk, too, although for different reasons. (We'll discuss pediatric considerations in Section 4.) Other high-risk patients include those with kidney or liver conditions and those patients who are either underweight, overweight, or malnourished.

Note: Chemicals in processed foods and in the air can interact with medications. Consider your patient at higher risk for drug interactions if he smokes or is routinely exposed to toxic fumes.

Your role. Minimizing the risks begins with a complete drug history. Keep in mind that your patient may himself be unsure of all the medications he's taking. If he can't name them all, ask him to describe them or ask a family member to bring them to the hospital. Alert the doctor to any potential problems you identify. *Note:* In some hospitals, the pharmacist is available to interview the patient about his medications.

Remember that proper patient teaching is just as important as a good drug history. Encourage the patient to treat all medications—including OTC products—with respect.

IDENTIFYING AN INTERACTION: NO EASY TASK

No one can remember all the possible interactions for all possible drug combinations. That's why you, the doctor, and the pharmacist must rely on reference books and other sources of drug information for help. But remember, not all interactions are textbook examples. Consider these variables:
• An interaction may not produce a reaction for several days.
• Individual differences in absorption, distribution, metabolism, and excretion rates can cause unexpected interactions in some patients.
• The patient and health-care professionals may mistakenly attribute an adverse reaction to the patient's medical condition rather than to a drug interaction.
• Some interactions depend on the order in which the drugs are given.

• An interaction may be mistaken for an adverse effect of a drug recently added to the regimen.

Undercover interaction. A recently discovered interaction between quinidine and digoxin illustrates the last example. Among the first cardiovascular drugs to be used clinically, quinidine and digoxin are commonly combined to treat atrial dysrhythmias; the pairing works effectively but may produce GI problems.

Digoxin is usually the first drug administered, with quinidine added later, if necessary. Since GI problems are a common adverse reaction to quinidine, health-care professionals once blamed the second drug for the discomfort.

But recent studies show that the GI problems have another cause: patients' plasma digoxin levels were doubling within a few days of the start of quinidine therapy, resulting in digoxin toxicity. Quinidine apparently alters tissue distribution and binding of digoxin and also decreases the amount of digoxin excreted.

That discovery opened the way to safe, effective use of the drug combination. Decreasing the digoxin dose when quinidine is introduced compensates for the interaction, allowing the percentage of active drug to stay at a therapeutic level.

How to cope. The drug interaction charts in Section 5 are designed to help you anticipate drug interactions. As you'll see, many interacting drugs can be given together safely, providing you take precautions. For example, you may adjust dosage (as ordered), monitor plasma drug levels, and closely monitor patient response.

LEARNING ABOUT DRUG INTERACTIONS 47

A.D.M.E.

How drug interactions affect drug processing

When the doctor prescribes a drug for your patient, he expects its absorption, distribution, metabolism, and excretion to follow a predictable pattern. But another drug that's already in the patient's system may interfere with the usual operation of those four processes, possibly strengthening, weakening, or negating the new drug's effect.

You already understand, from information in this book's second section, how a drug travels through a patient's system. After reading this section, you'll understand the ways one drug can alter another's usual passage. Because these interactions affect absorption, distribution, metabolism, and excretion, we'll use the acronym A.D.M.E. to describe any interaction of this type.

We'll also discuss how the planned use of some interactions can aid therapy and why the unplanned occurrence of others can cause setbacks. Your developing awareness may enable you to alert a busy doctor about a possible interaction that he might not have considered.

How interactions affect G.I. tract absorption

The most significant interactions affecting drug absorption involve orally administered drugs as they pass through the GI tract. For the most part, these interactions affect the *rate* of absorption, although the amount of absorption is also affected in some circumstances.

Motility and physiochemical changes caused by drugs play the biggest role in absorption interactions. For details, read on.

Motility. The degree of GI motility affects both the rate and amount of drug absorption. A drug that increases motility (for example, metoclopramide hydrochloride) can increase the absorption *rate* of rapidly dissolving drugs, such as acetaminophen. But it can decrease the *amount* of absorption by moving the drug through the GI tract too quickly.

Similarly, drugs that slow motility (narcotics and anticholinergics, for example) influence absorption by prolonging gastric emptying time. By slowing gastric emptying, these drugs improve the absorption of acidic drugs, which are normally absorbed from the stomach. Likewise, they delay the absorption of basic drugs, which are normally absorbed from the small intestine. But because slow motility allows these drugs to stay in the small intestine longer than usual, complete absorption eventually occurs.

When assessing how an interaction influencing GI motility will affect your patient, consider two factors: where the drug is normally absorbed and your patient's condition.

Physiochemical changes. Alterations in GI tract pH can affect absorption by influencing drug ionization. You'll recall that nonionized drugs readily penetrate lipid membranes, like those of the GI tract. Any drug that alters the pH of the GI tract changes the absorption pattern for a drug taken later. If the patient takes an antacid, for example, his normally acidic gastric fluid becomes more alkaline. As a result, any weak-base drug he ingests will remain nonionized and can be quickly absorbed. But a weak-acid drug, which is normally absorbed in the stomach, is likely to become so highly ionized that it's poorly absorbed in the stomach. But most of the ionized drug will probably be absorbed in the small intestine because of its large surface area. (For examples of weak-acid and weak-base drugs, see the chart on the opposite page.)

Changes in gastric pH can also affect drug dissolution. If a patient takes an enteric-coated tablet shortly after taking an antacid, the tablet's coating will dissolve in the stomach instead of the small intestine, possibly causing gastric irritation. This premature dissolution may also lead to intensified drug effects from the unusually rapid absorption.

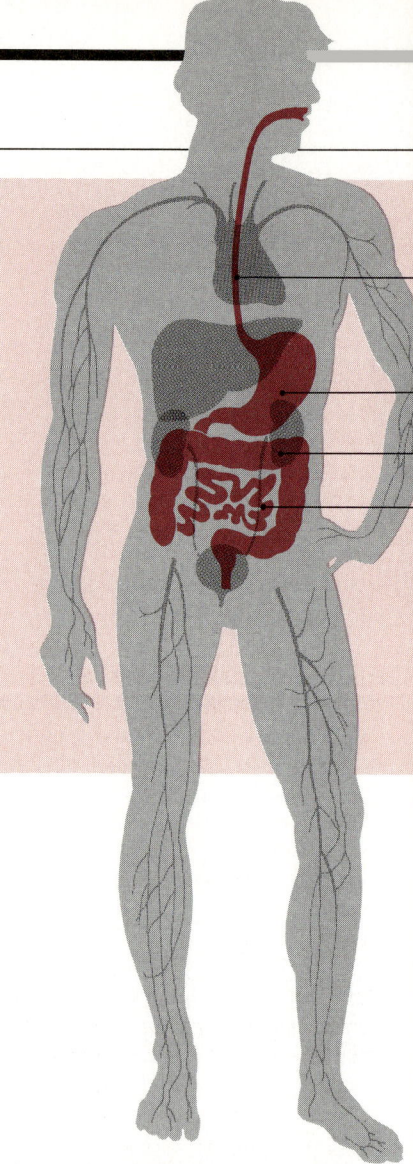

48 LEARNING ABOUT DRUG INTERACTIONS

GI Absorption

Esophagus

Stomach

Large intestine

Small intestine

Orally administered drugs have the greatest potential for absorption interactions. Because each portion of the GI tract absorbs drugs differently, factors affecting absorption—intestinal motility and pH, for example—vary in significance throughout the GI tract.

ACIDS AND BASES: A FEW EXAMPLES

WEAK ACIDS	WEAK BASES
Aspirin	Amitriptyline
Barbiturates	Amphetamines
Cephalosporins	Antihistamines
Ibuprofen	Antimalarials
Indomethacin	Cardiac depressants
Nalidixic acid	Diazepam
Penicillins	Ephedrine
Phenylbutazone	Morphine and derivatives
Phenytoin	Phenothiazine antipsychotics
Probenecid	Physostigmine and analogs
Sulfonamides	Quinine and quinidine
Thyroxine	Reserpine
Warfarin	

RATE VERSUS AMOUNT

How much drug enters the bloodstream is always important. How quickly it enters usually isn't. But absorption rate *does* demand consideration when:
• reaching peak level rapidly is necessary for maximum effect (as with analgesics, psychotropics, antibiotics, or antiarrhythmics).
• delaying absorption may cause the drug's effects to last too long (a risk with some sedatives).
• relieving acute symptoms is the primary purpose of treatment.

DRUG COMPLEXES: AN ABSORPTION PROBLEM

For most drugs, a change in the patient's intestinal pH presents only a temporary obstacle. The intended amount of drug reaches the patient's bloodstream eventually, though more slowly than usual.

For a few interacting drugs, though, the total amount absorbed is decreased—because the drugs form complexes that are poorly absorbed. The result of this process, called *complexation*, is that most of the drug never reaches the intended receptors.

Tetracycline, for instance, forms complexes when given with aluminum, magnesium, or calcium. So, if the patient takes tetracycline with milk (or any milk product), little of the drug will take effect. (Newer types of tetracycline—doxycycline and minocycline—apparently don't form complexes with milk or food, but they do with aluminum hydroxide gel.)

Timing can solve many problems with complexation. Giving tetracycline 1 hour before an antacid usually allows enough time for drug absorption.

Note: Complexation can be exploited for beneficial effects. Some sustained-release and prolonged-action medications, for example, are designed to employ complexation to extend the drug's duration of action.

COMPETITIVE BINDING AND DISTRIBUTION

The drug-interaction risks your patient faces don't end with successful absorption. During distribution, an interaction between two drugs with an affinity for the same plasma proteins can cause serious problems.

As you'll remember, not all of a drug's molecules immediately bind to receptor sites for action. Some bind to plasma proteins instead. This bound drug/free drug ratio normally stays constant as long as the drug remains in the system: metabolism and excretion remove free-drug molecules from the system, and plasma proteins release enough molecules to take their place.

Binding-site competition. When a second drug enters the system, problems may arise. If the new drug has a higher affinity for the sites occupied by the first drug, some displacement occurs. Molecules of the new drug knock the earlier drug off some binding sites, making a higher-than-normal percentage of the first drug available to receptors. As a result, the displaced drug's effect intensifies because more drug is active in the patient's system. But paradoxically, the drug's duration of action *shortens*, because more free-drug molecules are available for metabolism more quickly.

Assessing the danger. Not all drug displacements are hazardous. Some are almost negligible in their effect. Most problems occur when the displaced drug is normally at least 90% bound. Why? Because even a small increase of free drug means a large increase in the active amount. Also, highly bound drugs are usually highly potent.

But drugs don't necessarily pose a problem just because

CONTINUED ON PAGE 50

A.D.M.E.

COMPETITIVE BINDING AND DISTRIBUTION CONTINUED
they're highly bound. Digitoxin, for instance, is highly bound, and no other drug displaces it significantly.

The drugs that can displace one another, possibly causing serious adverse effects, include sulfa drugs, phenylbutazone, tolbutamide, and anticoagulants. Which drug displaces another drug depends largely on the concentrations of each present.

Other factors that can enhance or diminish one drug's ability to displace others include the following.
• Increased dosage levels tend to make a drug more effective as a displacer; some drugs become displacers only when given in large doses.
• A drug given with two other drugs that compete with it for the same plasma proteins may be able to displace the more weakly bound drug, without disturbing the more highly bound drug.

Calculating for displacement. The fact that two drugs compete for the same proteins doesn't necessarily mean they can never be used together—but it does signal the need for careful monitoring when they are. Quinidine, for instance, apparently displaces digoxin. But, as you learned on page 47, quinidine/digoxin therapy works safely and effectively when only about half the normal digoxin dose is given with quinidine.

Similar adjustments can make other combinations workable—as long as the prescribing doctor makes another dosage adjustment when one of the interacting drugs is stopped. Remember, the remaining drug will revert to its earlier binding characteristics, possibly changing the level of active drug in the patient's bloodstream.

Distribution
After absorption into the bloodstream, some drugs bind to plasma proteins and others remain free. Both free- and bound-drug molecules are distributed to tissue throughout the body; free molecules then bind to receptor sites. During this process, two or more drugs may compete for protein binding sites or receptor sites.

Compensation—the safety valve. When an excess of free drug is circulating, the body works to metabolize and eliminate the extra molecules, so that bound drug/free drug levels return to normal as soon as possible. The greater the drug's apparent volume of distribution, the more quickly compensation occurs—sometimes so quickly that the patient experiences no adverse reaction. However, if the displaced drug is a highly bound, narrowly distributed drug that requires metabolism for inactivation, serious problems can occur—particularly in patients with hepatic or renal problems.

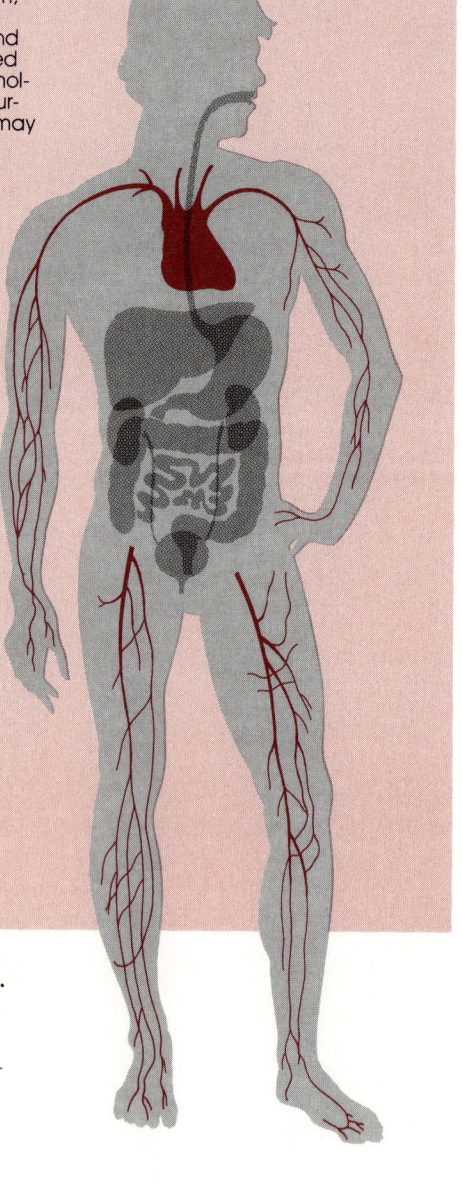

RECOGNIZING DRUG DISPLACERS

The following drugs (or, in a few cases, their metabolites) are among the most likely to displace other drugs from plasma protein-binding sites.

- Barbiturates
- Chloral hydrate
- Clofibrate
- Diazoxide
- Ethacrynic acid
- Hypoglycemics (oral)
- Indomethacin
- Mefenamic acid
- Nalidixic acid
- Oxyphenbutazone
- Phenylbutazone
- Phenytoin sodium
- Salicylates
- Sulfinpyrazone
- Sulfonamides
- Triiodothyronine

METABOLISM INTERACTIONS

When a drug reaches its receptor sites, half its journey is still ahead. The next stage, metabolism, is where drug interactions frequently occur.

You'll remember that metabolism occurs as a result of the action of an enzyme (in the case of drugs, usually a microsomal enzyme produced in the liver). Drug interactions at this stage involve either *enzyme induction* or *enzyme inhibition:* a drug may either speed or slow the liver's production of enzymes that act on newly introduced drugs.

Along with alcohol and nicotine, anticonvulsants (including barbiturates, carbamazepine, and phenytoin) *cause* significant metabolic changes. In contrast, these drug types may be *affected by* metabolic changes:
- oral anticoagulants
- oral antidiabetics
- steroids
- theophylline (because this has a very narrow therapeutic index, even minor changes are significant)
- tricyclic antidepressants.

Keeping the interactive potential of these drugs in mind should help you to be alert for early signs of metabolism problems.

CONTINUED ON PAGE 52

Metabolism
Liver

Most drug metabolism occurs in the liver (although the intestinal walls also metabolize some orally administered drugs). Orally administered drugs may undergo first-pass metabolism in the liver before reaching receptor sites. Other drugs are metabolized (usually into inactive metabolites) following distribution to receptor sites.

A.D.M.E.

METABOLISM INTERACTIONS CONTINUED

What happens in enzyme induction and enzyme inhibition to interfere with the body's handling of drugs? Let's take a look.

Enzyme induction. When a drug like phenobarbital stimulates the liver to increase enzyme production, metabolism occurs more quickly and shortens the active life of subsequently taken medications. While many drugs aren't given for a long enough time and in large enough doses to produce clinically significant enzyme induction, potent enzyme inducers like phenobarbital can markedly alter the body's response to other drugs. And the effects of an enzyme-inducing drug can persist for months after the patient stops taking it.

You'll remember that metabolism turns most active drugs into inactive ones (detoxifies them), but that a few drugs don't become active until they've been metabolized. Knowing this, you can understand why enzyme induction can be either helpful or dangerous. When it accelerates the transformation of hazardous chemicals to neutral substances, it can help reverse toxic effects. But when a drug's metabolites are active and/or more toxic than the parent drug, enzyme induction can burden the body with a high concentration of potentially harmful substances.

Enzyme induction poses a special hazard for women using oral contraceptives that contain low-dose estrogen. The amount of estrogen the pills contain is so small that even a slight increase in metabolism could cause drug concentration in the blood to drop below effective contraceptive levels. The enzyme-inducer rifampin has been shown to increase estrogen metabolism to this degree.

The polycyclic hydrocarbons present in cigarette smoke also act as enzyme inducers. They may speed the metabolism of some drugs, such as theophylline and diazepam, making their dosage requirements somewhat greater.

Enzyme inhibition. Now, suppose one drug prevents the production of enzymes necessary for the metabolism of a second drug. In this case, a higher-than-normal level of unmetabolized molecules from the second drug circulates. This may exaggerate the drug's effect. And, since most drugs can't be excreted until metabolism changes them to an inactive, water-soluble form, excess drug molecules remain in the body longer. Duration of action increases—and the drug has greater potential to cause toxicity. For example, cimetidine inhibits the metabolism of diazepam, prolonging diazepam's effect.

Compensating for interactions. Some drugs causing metabolic interactions can be used together—carefully. If, for instance, a patient on warfarin begins to take phenobarbital, which stimulates warfarin metabolism, his anticoagulant level will drop. The doctor will probably increase the warfarin dosage to compensate. But if the doctor later discontinues phenobarbital, the patient will again metabolize warfarin normally. His prothrombin time will rise—and, unless the doctor cuts warfarin back to the earlier level, the patient could hemorrhage.

Note: Warfarin levels may remain high for several days, until the excess is metabolized.

As always, patient teaching is essential. Teach the patient to take all drugs precisely as prescribed. Remember, noncompliance can diminish the effectiveness of drug therapy and exacerbate the patient's condition.

USING ENZYME INHIBITION AND INDUCTION

Like most drug interactions, those affecting metabolism are most dangerous when least expected. Deliberate, planned changes in metabolic rate, on the other hand, can be used therapeutically. Here are two examples.

• Treatment for alcoholism may include daily use of disulfiram (Antabuse), an enzyme inhibitor. Normally, alcohol undergoes two-stage metabolism: first to acetaldehyde and then to carbon dioxide and water. Disulfiram, which remains effective for at least 12 hours after ingestion, prevents the second metabolic step. If a person who has taken disulfiram ingests alcohol—even the minute amount in some cough syrups—toxic levels of acetaldehyde build up in his body, causing nausea, vomiting, headache, and other highly unpleasant effects.

• Although used infrequently, enzyme induction can help correct hyperbilirubinemia in newborns. This condition results from any number of problems, including hemolytic and hepatic disorders, that create a buildup of unmetabolized bilirubin in body tissues. Administering phenobarbital stimulates the newborn's liver to produce additional enzymes to metabolize the bilirubin, averting the damage that could develop from its accumulation in the brain. (Because phototherapy corrects hyperbilirubinemia more quickly than enzyme induction, it's now the preferred treatment.)

EXCRETION INTERACTIONS

The final stage in a drug's journey through the body, the excretion process strongly influences drug action. Consequently, any factor affecting this process also contributes to drug interactions.

Because the kidneys are the most important route for drug excretion, we'll focus on urinary excretion here. But keep in mind that factors affecting fecal excretion can be significant, too. For example, cathartics can reduce absorption of orally administered drugs by increasing GI motility. Factors affecting the excretion of drugs in sweat, saliva, tears, bile, and breast milk are relatively unimportant to the patient. (Of course, drug excretion in breast milk, even if minute, can have a significant effect on a nursing infant.)

You'll recall that urinary excretion involves glomerular filtration, tubular secretion, and reabsorption of substances from urine. Filtration is a passive process, and no significant changes in filtration occur from drug interactions. But, for the other two processes, drug interactions can make a difference. Let's consider them one at a time.

Tubular secretion. Tubular secretion, you'll recall, is an active transport process, meaning that molecules rely on active transport mechanisms to carry them across the membranes into the renal tubules. Any interaction that affects active transport mechanisms also affects tubular drug secretion.

The interaction between probenecid and penicillin provides an example. Probenecid competes with penicillin for transport, blocking the excretion of penicillin. Because penicillin remains in the body longer, its effects are prolonged.

This process, called *competi-*

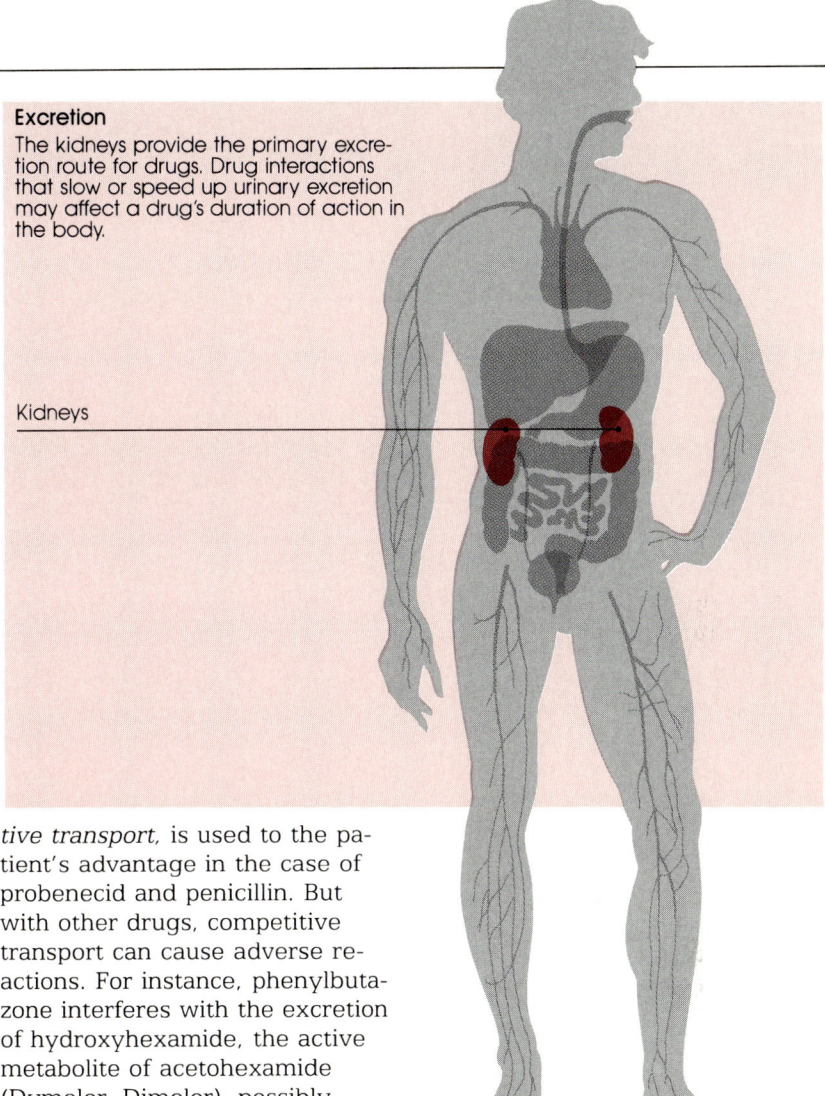

Excretion
The kidneys provide the primary excretion route for drugs. Drug interactions that slow or speed up urinary excretion may affect a drug's duration of action in the body.

Kidneys

tive transport, is used to the patient's advantage in the case of probenecid and penicillin. But with other drugs, competitive transport can cause adverse reactions. For instance, phenylbutazone interferes with the excretion of hydroxyhexamide, the active metabolite of acetohexamide (Dymelor, Dimelor), possibly causing hypoglycemia.

Tubular reabsorption. Ionized drugs are the easiest for the body to excrete. As you learned on page 26, environmental pH affects ionization: weak-acid drugs in urine become more highly ionized (and therefore are more readily excreted) in high-pH (alkaline) urine. Conversely, weak-base drugs are more highly ionized in low-pH (acidic) urine. A drug that increases the ionization of another traps the second drug in urine and accelerates its elimination. A drug that decreases ionization makes the second drug easier to reabsorb from urine into the circulation, so its plasma levels remain higher for a longer period. For example, antacids enhance the reabsorption of quinidine by raising urine pH.

Other factors. Any drug, condition, or process that alters urinary output may also affect drug excretion. Diuretics, for example, speed up excretion by increasing the glomerular filtration rate. This, in turn, speeds the excretion of other drugs the patient's taking. Similarly, drugs or pathologic conditions that damage nephrons diminish the kidneys' ability to excrete drugs.

LEARNING ABOUT DRUG INTERACTIONS 53

RECEPTOR-SITE ACTION

UNDERSTANDING RECEPTOR-SITE INTERACTIONS

On the preceding pages, we discussed how drug interactions can affect drug absorption, distribution, metabolism, and excretion. Now, let's see how drug interactions can affect drug action at receptor sites.

During distribution, drug molecules travel to receptor sites, which trigger the drug's therapeutic effect. When two drugs enter the body, they may contact the same receptor site simultaneously and compete for it. Depending on the specific drugs and the patient's condition, this competition for a receptor site can increase or decrease the therapeutic effectiveness of one or both drugs. In some cases, the result is a potentially hazardous interaction; in others, an enhancement of therapy that benefits the patient.

Receptor-site interactions may be additive, synergistic, or antagonistic. Read what follows for examples of each type.

ADDITIVE INTERACTIONS: WHEN ONE PLUS ONE EQUALS TWO

When you simultaneously administer drugs that produce similar effects, one drug can add to the effect of the other drug. The resulting interaction is *additive,* or equal to the sum of the drugs' separate effects. This additive effect isn't necessarily adverse; in fact, additive interactions are a cornerstone of combination drug therapy. But *unplanned* additive interactions can be dangerous. Consider the following examples of beneficial and adverse additive interactions.

Beneficial interactions. Suppose your patient is taking codeine for postoperative pain. When the codeine doesn't control the patient's pain, the doctor prescribes aspirin in conjunction with the codeine. Taken separately, each drug produces pain relief. But when taken together, the two drugs relieve pain about twice as well.

Codeine and acetaminophen also interact to cause additive analgesic effects. To take advantage of this therapeutic interaction, the doctor may order a combination product, such as Tylenol With Codeine No. 3*.

An adverse interaction. In contrast, suppose your patient's taking an antianxiety drug, such as prazepam (Centrax*). When the patient develops an allergic reaction to an insect sting, the doctor prescribes diphenhydramine hydrochloride (Benadryl), an antihistamine. Taken separately, prazepam and diphenhydramine each cause mild sedation. But when taken together, the drugs may produce extreme sedation. In this case, you'll warn the patient to avoid driving and other activities requiring alertness.

SYNERGISTIC INTERACTIONS: WHEN ONE PLUS ONE EQUALS FOUR

A *synergistic* interaction occurs when one drug potentiates (multiplies) the effects of another drug. In contrast to an additive interaction, synergism produces an effect *greater* than the sum of the drugs' separate effects.

In certain circumstances, you may not be able to identify whether an interaction is additive or synergistic. For example, alcohol and diazepam interact to increase sedation. But pharmacists debate whether this interaction is additive or synergistic.

As with additive interactions, synergism can have either beneficial or adverse effects.

A beneficial interaction. You're probably familiar with the antibiotic co-trimoxazole (Bactrim, Septra). Drug manufacturers developed co-trimoxazole, a combination of sulfamethoxazole and trimethoprim, to take advantage of the synergistic interaction between these two antibiotics. When prescribed separately, each merely inhibits bacterial growth. But, when given together as co-trimoxazole, they interact synergistically to kill bacteria.

An adverse interaction. Conversely, synergism can result in an adverse interaction that is greater than the sum of its parts. For example, aminoglycosides and furosemide (Lasix) each can cause ototoxicity when given separately. However, when both drugs are given to a patient, the possibility of his developing ototoxicity increases tremendously. This synergistic ototoxic effect can produce permanent hearing loss.

*Not available in Canada

ELECTROLYTES

ANTAGONISTIC INTERACTIONS: WHEN ONE PLUS ONE EQUALS ZERO

Certain drugs, when given simultaneously, *antagonize* one another. In other words, one drug blocks the other drug's effectiveness, negating any therapeutic value.

A beneficial interaction. Suppose your postoperative patient complains of pain. You administer the narcotic meperidine hydrochloride (Demerol), as ordered. Subsequently, his respiration drops sharply and you can't arouse him. So, as ordered, you administer a narcotic antagonist, such as naloxone hydrochloride (Narcan). The antagonist reverses the narcotic's effects, and the patient's level of consciousness and respiratory rate improve. Of course, the antagonist also reverses the narcotic's analgesic effects, so the patient's pain returns.

Adverse interactions. On the other hand, an unanticipated antagonistic interaction can prevent an intended therapeutic effect from occurring. For example, suppose a patient taking propranolol hydrochloride (Inderal) for hypertension is given albuterol (Proventil*) to relieve an asthma attack. Normally, albuterol relieves bronchospasm by dilating the bronchi. But, as you'll recall, one of propranolol's usual effects is to *constrict* the bronchi. Thus, if these two drugs are given together, their opposing effects on the bronchi counteract each other, depriving the patient of albuterol's intended therapeutic effect. For this reason, propranolol and albuterol shouldn't be given together.

The interaction between warfarin and vitamin K is another example. Vitamin K antagonizes warfarin, reversing its anticoagulant effect.

*Not available in Canada

HOW ELECTROLYTE IMBALANCES AFFECT DRUG THERAPY

When considering factors that may affect your patient's response to drug therapy, don't neglect to assess his electrolyte values. By controlling the body's fluid and chemical balance, electrolytes inevitably affect drug action. Consequently, any electrolyte imbalance increases the risk of an adverse reaction that otherwise might not occur. Read the following chart for a review of electrolyte imbalances and how they affect drug therapy.

POTASSIUM

Normal levels: 3.5 to 5.0 mEq/liter. This major intracellular cation (positively charged ion) aids many enzyme reactions, helps regulate acid-base balance, maintains normal neuromuscular excitability, and helps transport glucose into cells.

HYPOKALEMIA

Possible causes include gastric fluid loss from vomiting or diarrhea; diuretic therapy; therapy with glucocorticoids, amphotericin B, or carbenicillin; kidney disease, such as nephritis or renal tubular necrosis; and excessive diaphoresis.

Signs and symptoms
• Anorexia, nausea, vomiting
• Muscle weakness, eventually leading to paralysis and respiratory arrest
• Drowsiness, confusion, central nervous system (CNS) irritability
• Cardiac dysrhythmias
• EKG changes, such as depressed ST segments, flat or inverted T waves, and prominent U waves
• Bradycardia

Nursing considerations
• Hypokalemia increases the heart's sensitivity to digitalis. When administering digitalis to a hypokalemic patient—especially an elderly patient—monitor his potassium and digoxin or digitoxin levels, and watch for signs of toxicity. If the patient's also receiving amphotericin B, or any other drug which may cause hypokalemia, remember that this further increases the risk of digitalis toxicity.
• Potassium-losing diuretics, amphotericin B, corticosteroids, cathartics, and insulin can cause potassium depletion. Watch your hypokalemic patient closely if he's receiving any of these drugs. Monitor his intake and output and serum potassium level, and watch for EKG changes and other signs indicating potassium depletion. Also, adjust his diet to insure adequate potassium intake, and administer potassium supplements as ordered.
• Hypokalemia antagonizes the antiarrhythmic action of phenytoin, procainamide, lidocaine, and quinidine. Watch your hypokalemic patient closely if he's receiving any of these drugs.

HYPERKALEMIA

Possible causes of hyperkalemia include infections, Addison's disease, renal failure, prolonged treatment with potassium supplements, and therapy with potassium-sparing diuretics or captopril.

Signs and symptoms
• Muscle weakness, possibly leading to paralysis
• Neuromuscular hyperexcitability
• EKG changes, such as peaked T waves, depressed ST segments, and widened QRS complexes; possibly cardiac arrest

Nursing considerations
• Potassium-sparing diuretics (such as spironolactone, triamterene, and amiloride hydrochloride) can exacerbate hyperkalemia by increasing potassium levels. If your patient's receiving these drugs, watch for signs of worsening hyperkalemia. *Caution:* If your hyperkalemic patient's receiving

CONTINUED ON PAGE 56

ELECTROLYTES

HOW ELECTROLYTE IMBALANCES AFFECT DRUG THERAPY CONTINUED

potassium-sparing diuretics, give him potassium supplements cautiously, if at all. The combination may be life-threatening.
• Many forms of penicillin contain potassium. If your hyperkalemic patient's receiving one of these penicillin forms, monitor his potassium levels closely.
• Hyperkalemia can decrease digitalis' effectiveness. If your hyperkalemic patient's taking digitalis, watch for signs of heart failure or other indications that his cardiac condition is worsening.

MAGNESIUM

Normal levels: 1.5 to 2.5 mEq/liter. Like potassium, magnesium is an intracellular cation. Usually supplied by the diet, magnesium aids various enzyme reactions, which influences the metabolism of nucleic acids, proteins, and carbohydrates; helps regulate intracellular calcium levels; and affects the rate of neuromuscular impulse transmission throughout the CNS.

HYPOMAGNESEMIA

Possible causes include impaired intestinal absorption from chronic diarrhea or bowel resection, excessive renal excretion from diuretic therapy or alcoholism, malnutrition, cisplatin therapy, and acute pancreatitis.

Signs and symptoms
• Anorexia
• Muscle weakness
• Muscle spasticity
• Tremors, fasciculations
• Confusion, disorientation
• CNS irritability, convulsions
• EKG changes, such as prolonged QT intervals and small, broad T waves

Nursing consideration
• Hypomagnesemia increases the heart's sensitivity to digitalis. If your patient's receiving digitalis, watch him closely for signs of digitalis toxicity.

HYPERMAGNESEMIA

Possible causes of hypermagnesemia include chronic renal failure; excessive use of antacids or cathartics containing magnesium, such as Epsom salt and milk of magnesia; adrenal insufficiency; and prolonged magnesium therapy.

Signs and symptoms
With serum magnesium levels from 2.6 to 3.0 mEq/liter:
• None
With serum magnesium levels from 3.1 to 5.0 mEq/liter:
• Nausea, vomiting
• Hypotension
• Depressed deep-tendon reflexes
With serum magnesium levels from 5.1 to 7.0 mEq/liter:
• Depressed deep-tendon reflexes
• Drowsiness
• Depression
With serum magnesium levels from 7.1 to 10.0 mEq/liter:
• Weakness
• Loss of deep-tendon reflexes
• Sinus bradycardia
• EKG changes, such as prolonged PR intervals and QT intervals
With serum magnesium levels from 10.1 to 15.0 mEq/liter:
• Paralysis
• Coma
• Hypoventilation
With serum magnesium levels from 15.1 to 20.0 mEq/liter:
• Apnea
• Cardiac arrest

Nursing considerations
• Administering magnesium sulfate to a hypermagnesemic patient with pregnancy-induced hypertension can be fatal. *Use extreme caution.*
• Renal failure prevents magnesium excretion. If your patient has renal failure, avoid giving drugs that contain magnesium, including such antacids as Maalox Plus and Mylanta.

CALCIUM

Normal levels: 8.5 to 10.5 mg/100 ml. Calcium, like magnesium, is supplied by diet. Dependent on vitamin D for absorption, calcium is essential for bone formation. It also helps regulate enzyme systems, aids in metabolism, enables muscles to contract, influences transmission of neuromuscular impulses, and influences blood coagulation.

HYPOCALCEMIA

Possible causes include hypoparathyroidism, vitamin D deficiency, inadequate calcium intake, and renal failure.

Signs and symptoms
• Nausea, vomiting, diarrhea
• Muscle cramps
• Numbness and tingling of extremities
• Positive Chvostek's and Trousseau's signs
• Seizures
• Hyperreflexia
• Mental depression
• EKG changes, such as prolonged QT intervals and inverted T waves

Nursing considerations
• Corticosteroids decrease calcium absorption, causing calcium levels to drop. If your hypocalcemic patient's taking corticosteroids, check his calcium level regularly and adjust his dietary calcium intake if necessary.

56 LEARNING ABOUT DRUG INTERACTIONS

- Phosphates and loop diuretics promote calcium excretion. If your patient's taking either of these drugs, check his calcium level regularly.

HYPERCALCEMIA
Possible causes include primary hyperparathyroidism, vitamin A or D intoxication, prolonged use of certain antacids, and metastatic carcinomas.

Signs and symptoms
- Nausea, vomiting, anorexia
- Constipation
- Muscle weakness, fatigue
- Muscle hypotonicity
- Increased myocardial contractility
- Pathologic fractures
- Confusion, lethargy
- EKG changes, such as shortened QT intervals and appearance of U waves

Nursing consideration
- Hypercalcemia increases the heart's sensitivity to digitalis. If your patient's taking digitalis, watch him closely for signs of digitalis toxicity.

NEUROMUSCULAR IMPULSES: POTASSIUM'S ROLE

Potassium and other electrolytes—magnesium and calcium—transmit neuromuscular impulses. To see how, take a look at the illustration below.

During depolarization, sodium flows into the cell and potassium flows out. This electolyte exchange creates a positive electrical charge that stimulates neighboring cells to depolarize as well. Then the impulse spreads from cell to cell until a muscular contraction occurs. Once the signal is transmitted from a cell, the cell repolarizes, potassium flows back into the cell, and sodium flows out.

Any electrolyte disturbance disrupts this process by either delaying or accelerating impulses. For example, hypokalemia slows impulses, possibly disturbing the heart's normal rhythm and rate.

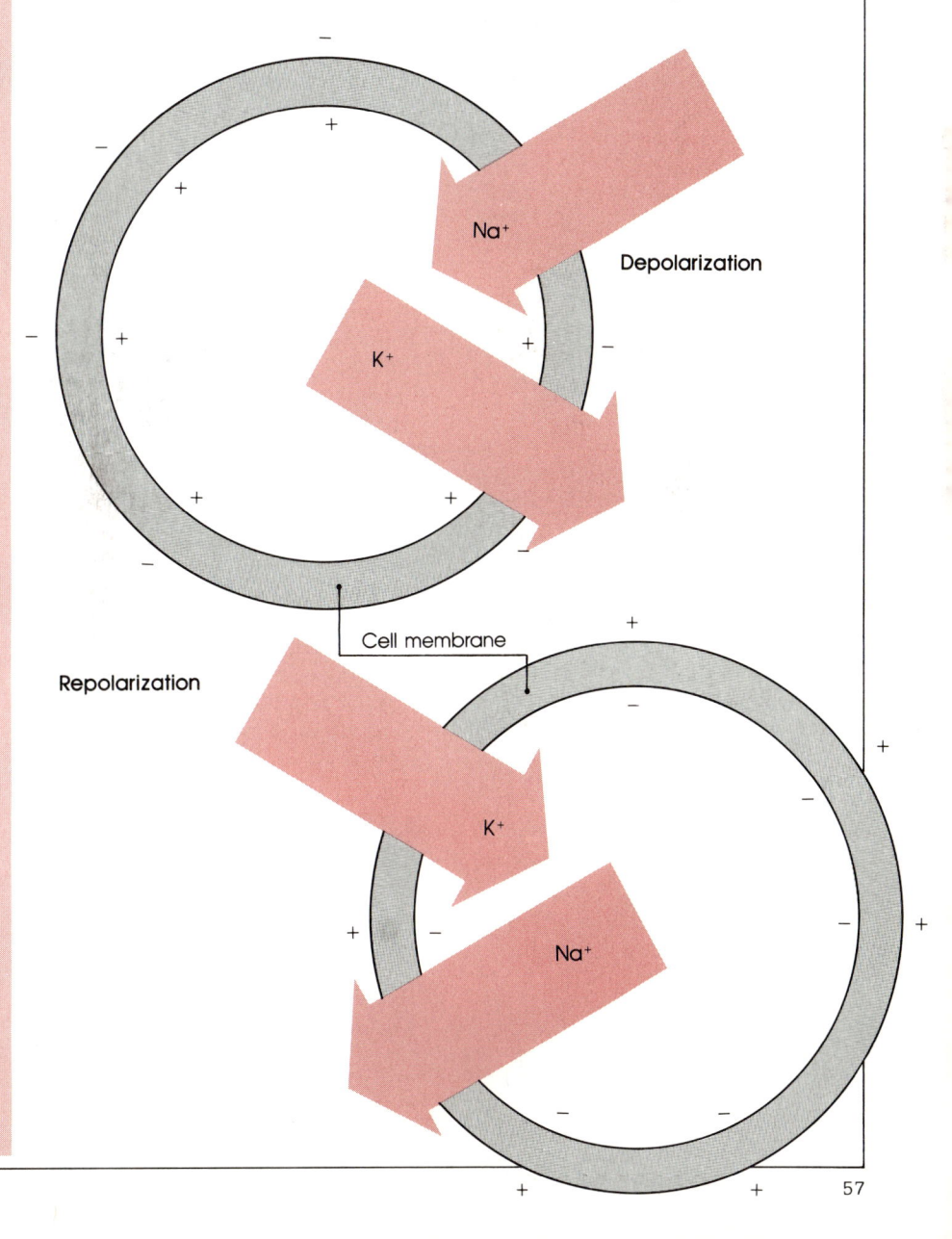

ELECTROLYTES

DRUG INTERACTIONS WITH ELECTROLYTES

The chart below lists several drugs and drug types that may affect your patient's potassium, magnesium, or calcium levels. Although these electrolyte level changes may be therapeutic in some instances, they can also place the patient at risk of a potentially dangerous electrolyte imbalance. If your patient's receiving any of these drugs, closely monitor his serum electrolyte levels and report imbalances.

DRUG	POSSIBLE EFFECTS
Acetazolamide	Hypocalcemia
Alcohol	Hypomagnesemia
Aminoglycosides	Hypomagnesemia, hypokalemia
Aminosalicylic acid	Hypokalemia
Amphotericin B	Hypokalemia, hypomagnesemia
Bumetanide	Hypomagnesemia, hypocalcemia, hypokalemia
Capreomycin	Hypomagnesemia, hypocalcemia
Cisplatin	Hypomagnesemia
Corticosteroids	Hypokalemia, hypocalcemia
Cycloserine	Hypomagnesemia, hypocalcemia
Dactinomycin	Hypocalcemia
Ethacrynic acid	Hypomagnesemia, hypocalcemia, hypokalemia
Furosemide	Hypomagnesemia, hypocalcemia, hypokalemia
Glutethimide	Hypocalcemia
Levodopa	Hypokalemia
Lithium	Hypermagnesemia, hypocalcemia
Mercurials	Hypomagnesemia, hypocalcemia
Oral contraceptives	Hypomagnesemia
Penicillins	Hypokalemia
Probenecid	Hypokalemia, hypomagnesemia, hypocalcemia
Salicylates	Hypokalemia
Spironolactone	Hypomagnesemia, hypocalcemia, hyperkalemia
Tetracyclines	Hypomagnesemia, hypocalcemia
Thiazides	Hypomagnesemia, hypercalcemia, hypokalemia
Triamterene	Hypocalcemia, hyperkalemia

YOUR ROLE

MINIMIZING INTERACTIONS: YOUR RESPONSIBILITY, TOO

Would you be surprised to learn that, according to one estimate, up to 25% of reported adverse reactions may actually be drug *interactions?* Such a finding (reported in the *Annals of Emergency Medicine,* December 1981) emphasizes that drug interactions are no small problem for healthcare professionals.

How does this affect you? While the doctor's responsible for prescribing drugs, *you're* responsible for administering them—and doing so safely. You can't expect to remember every potential interaction. But you can minimize risks by following these general safety guidelines:
• Take a thorough health history, including a drug history.
• Recognize patients at special risk of interactions—the young, the old, and those with certain chronic health problems, such as kidney or liver disease, congestive heart failure, or diabetes.
• Understand how drugs act and interact.
• Look up any drug you're not familiar with, and learn indications, contraindications, intended effects, and adverse effects. Some reference books include information on drug interactions, too.
• Call the pharmacist for more information, if necessary. Be sure to inform him about the patient's condition as well as the drug regimen.
• Watch out for drug administration errors. Use the Five Rights system, and take appropriate precautions if you find any discrepancies.

What else can you do to minimize your patient's risk? Read the following page for more tips.

GIVING HIGH-RISK DRUGS

The drugs most likely to interact dangerously with other drugs are those with narrow therapeutic indexes, such as theophylline. Drugs in the following categories are also likely to interact:
• oral anticoagulants
• antidiabetics
• cardiotonic glycosides
• cytotoxics
• anticonvulsants
• antihypertensives
• central nervous system (CNS) depressants.

Note: The GI drug cimetidine is considered a high-risk drug.

If your patient is taking other drugs, the doctor may try to replace a high-risk drug with a safer alternative. But if this isn't possible, take special care to keep the patient under close observation, monitor appropriate laboratory tests, and watch for any signs of drug toxicity or other adverse reactions.

ADMINISTRATION CONSIDERATIONS

Before you administer any drugs to your patient, consider these three administration factors:
• timing
• administration route
• order.

Each of these factors can affect a drug's potential for interaction. Here are a few examples.

Consider the timing. With some drug combinations, the timing of each drug dose is crucial. For such drugs, you can minimize interactions simply by spacing the doses apart.

Let's say, for instance, that your patient is currently receiving tetracycline and you want to give him an antacid for his heartburn. To avoid an interaction that may jeopardize antibiotic therapy, give tetracycline 2 hours after giving the antacid. Or give the antacid 1 hour after tetracycline. (If you give tetracycline first, be sure to tell your patient why you're waiting to give him the antacid.)

Consider the route. The administration route also influences a drug's potential to interact with other drugs. Drugs administered orally are most vulnerable to drug interactions. Unlike drugs administered intravenously, oral drugs must travel through the GI tract before being absorbed into the bloodstream. Other oral drugs administered simultaneously may interfere with the absorption process.

However, oral drugs aren't the only drugs susceptible to route-influenced interactions. For example, if you administer gentamicin and carbenicillin in the same I.V. infusion, the carbenicillin will destroy gentamicin's effectiveness. But, if you administer gentamicin intramuscularly and carbenicillin intravenously, they're less likely to interact.

Consider the order. A few drug interactions are influenced by the order in which you give the drugs. The interaction between tetracycline and penicillin is an example. Penicillin acts by inhibiting cell-wall synthesis (a bactericidal mechanism). Tetracycline, which inhibits protein synthesis (a bacteriostatic mechanism), can antagonize penicillin's bactericidal effect.

If possible, the doctor will avoid this combination. But if he can't, you can help minimize the interaction by administering penicillin at least 1 hour before tetracycline.

EVALUATING A NEW DRUG

Suppose you're asked to add another drug to your patient's regimen. You're unfamiliar with the drug and don't know if it will interact with other drugs your patient's receiving. Here's a brief checklist to help you evaluate the new drug's interaction potential.

• Is the drug highly protein-bound? If so, it may compete for protein-binding sites with another highly bound drug (such as warfarin or phenytoin). The patient may then experience exaggerated effects from one of the drugs.
• Is sedation a common adverse reaction? If so, the drug may cause additive or synergistic sedation if given with a CNS depressant.
• Does the drug cause hypotension? If so, it may cause additive hypotension if given with a nitrate or an antihypertensive drug.
• Does the drug affect the liver's enzyme activity? If so, it may accelerate or delay the metabolism of other drugs the patient's receiving, affecting their duration of action.

MODIFYING DRUG THERAPY

Administering drugs to a child? A pregnant woman? An elderly patient with a chronic kidney condition? Because all of these patients have conditions that complicate drug therapy, caring for them challenges your nursing skills.

Many patient factors, including age, genetic makeup, medical conditions, and life-style choices such as smoking and alcohol consumption, can alter drug action in the body. But exactly how these factors affect drug therapy varies. For example, GI disorders that cause vomiting and diarrhea reduce absorption of orally administered drugs, thus diminishing their effectiveness. On the other hand, liver disease may contribute to prolonged drug action by slowing drug metabolism.

Regardless of the circumstances, you're responsible for helping to make sure your patient receives the maximum benefit from drug therapy with minimal risk of adverse reactions. This section will help. You'll find sound and timely advice on how to ensure therapeutic results despite your patient's special problems.

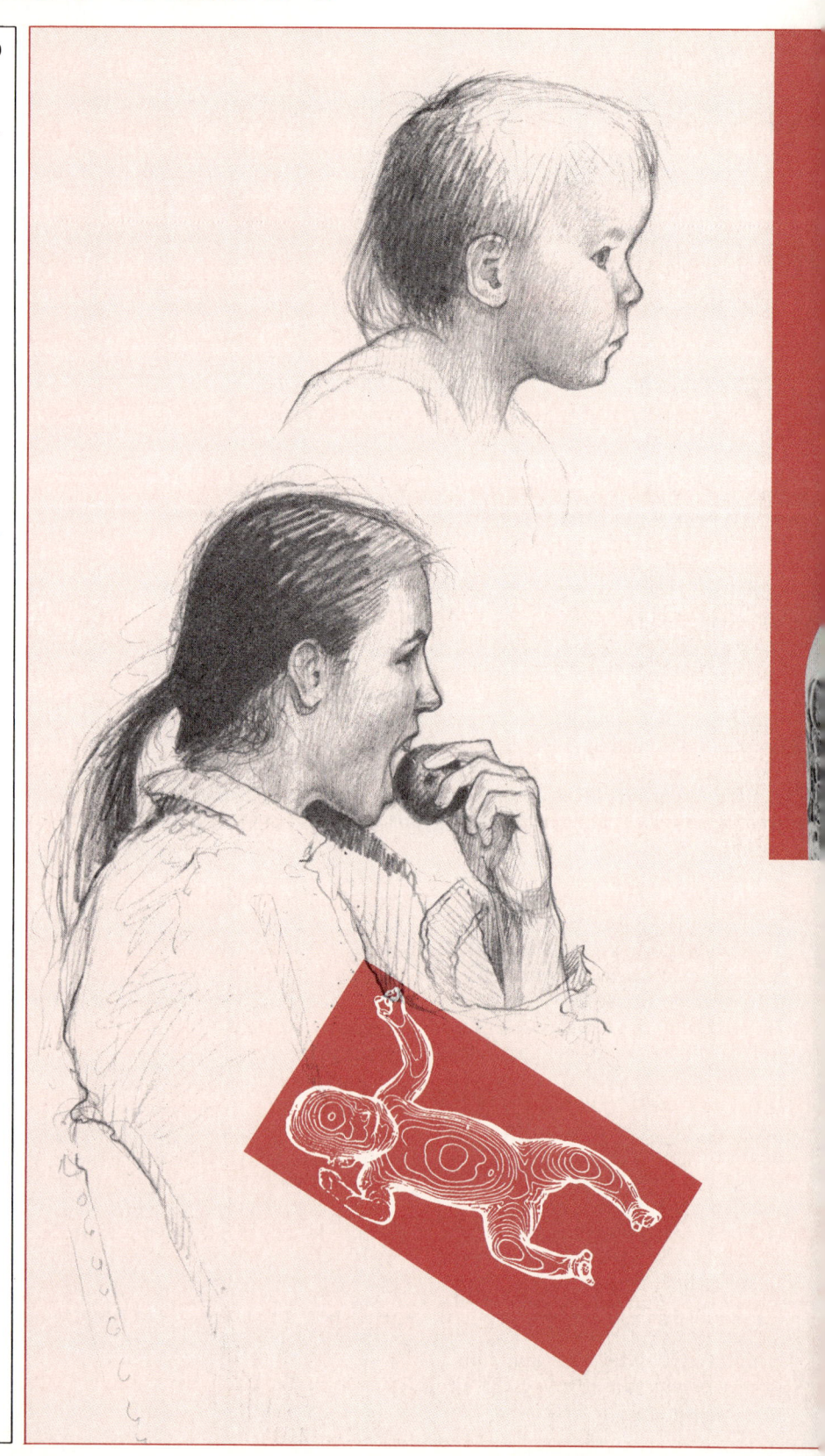

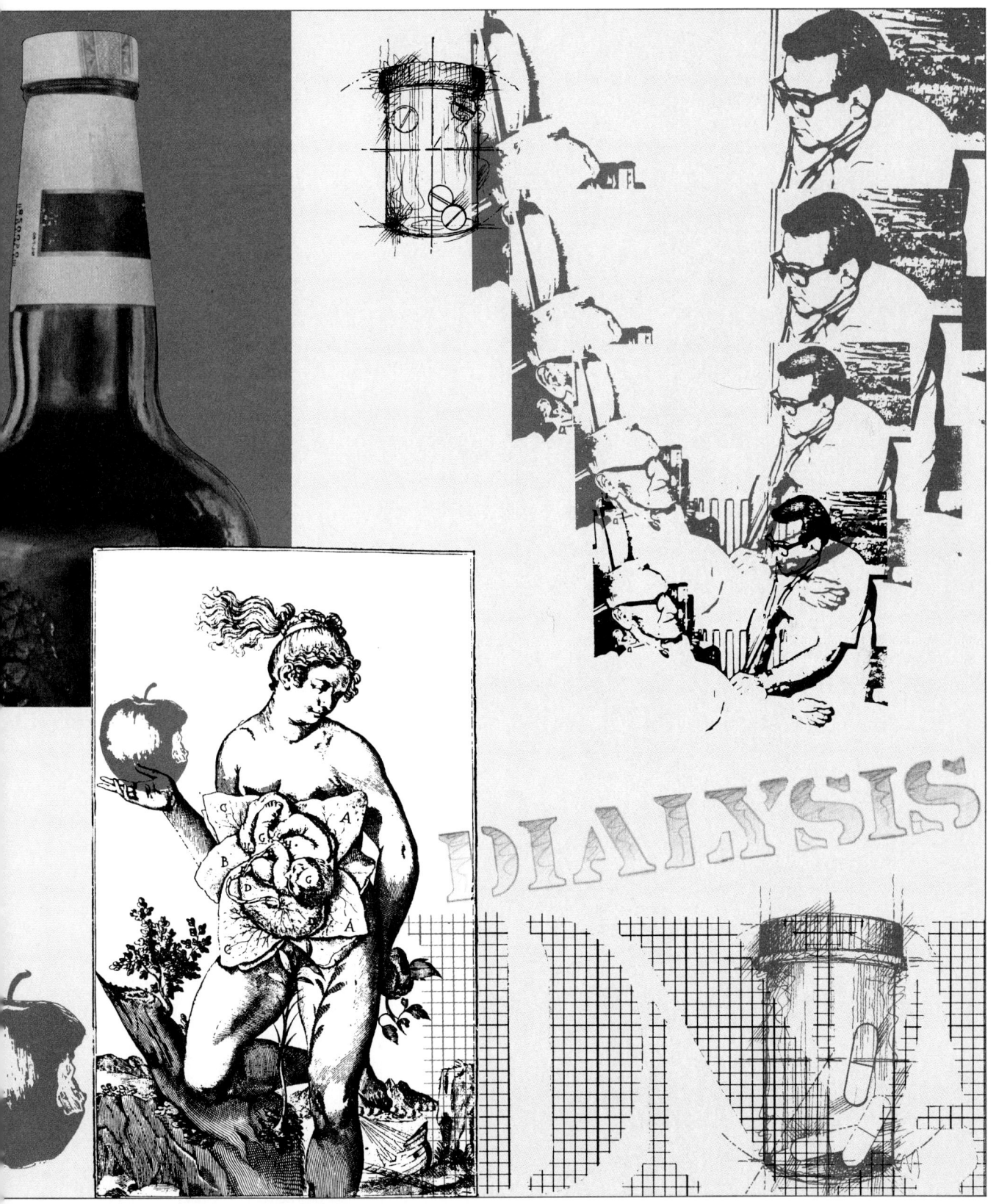

MODIFYING DRUG THERAPY

PREGNANCY

DRUGS AND THE PREGNANT PATIENT

Caring for a pregnant patient can be an exciting and rewarding experience. But when that patient has a health problem that requires drug therapy, caring for her becomes a special challenge for you. Any drug the mother takes, including over-the-counter products, alcohol, and illicit drugs, may cross the placenta and enter fetal circulation. In some cases, the effects of the drug on the fetus are negligible. In others, however, drug effects can have serious consequences. When given during the first trimester, for example, some drugs cause congenital abnormalities; in the third trimester, some drugs cause adverse reactions in the fetus or newborn. Although adverse drug reactions during the second trimester are not as well documented, drugs are known to cross the placenta and affect the fetus. That's why you should strongly advise your patient to avoid taking any drug preparation without her doctor's approval.

Important: Before administering drugs to any woman of childbearing age, be sure to rule out the possibility of pregnancy.

However, if drug therapy is absolutely necessary for your pregnant patient, administer the appropriate dosage with extreme caution and monitor the patient closely.

For a complete review of the action and implications of drugs in the pregnant patient, read this section carefully.

THE PREGNANT PATIENT: A UNIQUE TWOSOME

To safely and beneficially administer drugs to a pregnant patient, you must first understand the special nature of the maternal/fetal twosome. Because the physiology of mother and fetus is so closely intertwined, practically every substance that enters the mother's body eventually reaches the fetus in some form. Yet mother and fetus react to various substances, particularly drugs, in separate and distinct ways.

To care for both patients, you must be able to anticipate and accurately evaluate their individual responses to any drug the mother may take. Read what follows to learn how the basic physiology of pregnancy can alter drug action.

Maternal drug action. Several major physiologic changes occur in a pregnant woman that can interfere with drug action. First, a woman's blood and plasma volume increase to adequately vascularize the uterus and carry

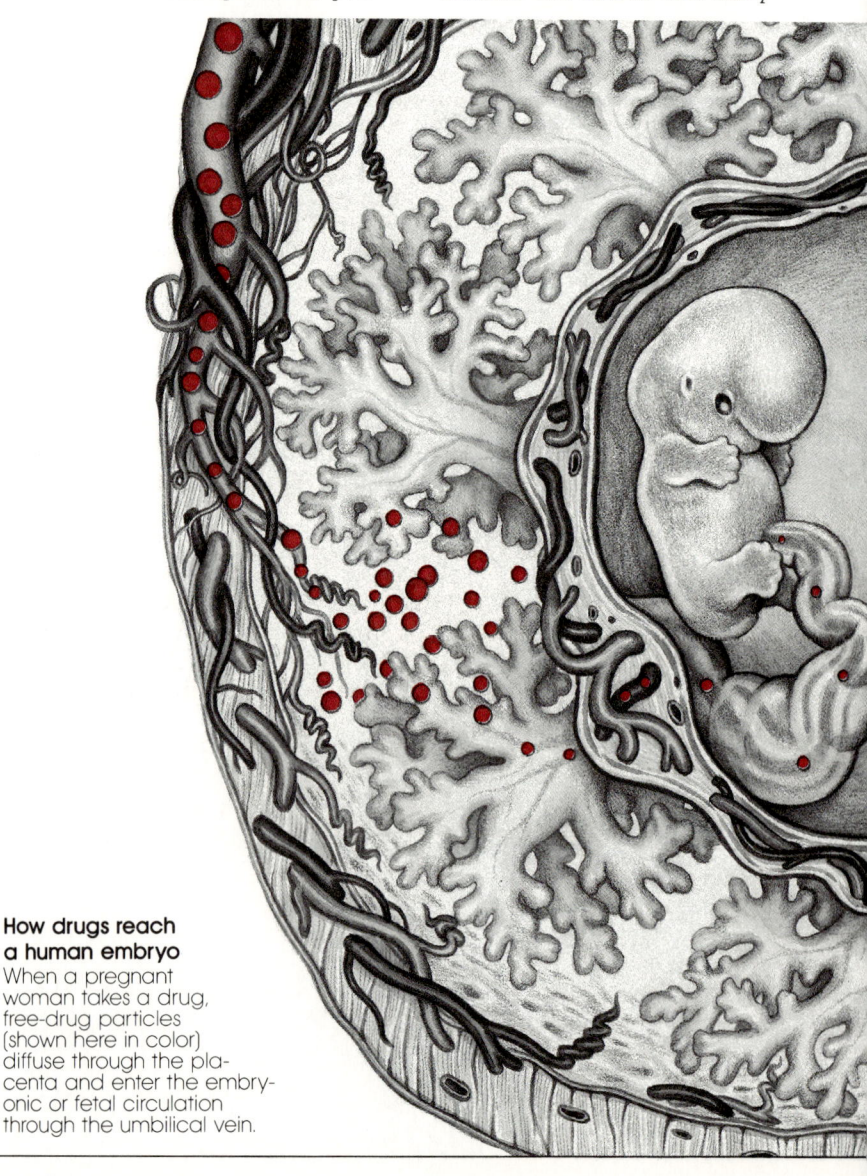

How drugs reach a human embryo
When a pregnant woman takes a drug, free-drug particles (shown here in color) diffuse through the placenta and enter the embryonic or fetal circulation through the umbilical vein.

sufficient nutrients and oxygen through the umbilical arteries to the fetus. Albumin production also increases during pregnancy. But since plasma volume expands to a greater degree, serum albumin concentration is proportionately lower. With less albumin available to bind drugs that enter the maternal system, more unbound, or free, drug is available to cross the placenta to the fetus.

In addition, because the pregnant woman's hepatic blood flow decreases, her liver metabolizes drugs more slowly than usual. Consequently, the transfer of unmetabolized drugs from mother to fetus occurs over a longer period of time, thus prolonging the drug's effect on the fetus.

On the other hand, renal blood flow and glomerular filtration *increase* during pregnancy, causing the woman's kidneys to excrete drugs more rapidly. As a result, you must carefully monitor drug dosage.

The placenta's role. Before a drug can reach the fetus, it must first cross the placental membrane. Any unbound, nonionized, lipid-soluble drug whose molecular weight is less than 1,000 can rapidly diffuse through any membrane. Since most drugs have a molecular weight of 250 to 500, simple diffusion is the mechanism that carries most drugs across the placental membrane.

Some drugs can't diffuse through the placenta without being broken down further. Placental enzymes metabolize these drugs, allowing them to enter the fetal circulation. Some drugs act as placental enzyme inducers, speeding drug transport to the fetus. In one way or another, and in one form or another, all drugs eventually reach the fetus.

Fetal drug action. Once a drug crosses the placenta and enters fetal circulation, it does one of two things, depending on its composition. The majority of drugs travel through the umbilical and portal veins to the fetal liver, where they're converted and detoxified. Although the process is much the same as in an adult, it occurs much more slowly.

Other drugs pass through the liver to the ductus venosus and inferior vena cava to the heart, which distributes the drugs to the brain and coronary arteries. Then, more than half of the blood and drug combination travels back through the umbilical arteries, crosses the placenta, and reenters maternal circulation. The remaining drug-laden blood continues to circulate in the fetus.

The fetus excretes the drug mainly through its kidneys. However, excretion is slow because of low renal blood flow, causing slow glomerular filtration and tubular absorption. Consequently, drugs may accumulate in the fetus.

The fetus excretes a small amount of drug through its lungs, sweat glands, and bile into the amniotic fluid. Because the fetus swallows the amniotic fluid, the excreted drugs are reabsorbed into the fetal circulation. This is another reason why fetal drug concentrations may be 50% to 100% higher than maternal drug concentrations.

CRITERIA FOR DRUG THERAPY
Because drug therapy for a pregnant patient places the fetus at risk for congenital abnormalities and other adverse reactions, drugs should be given to the mother only when absolutely necessary and only under close medical supervision.

Conditions for which drug therapy is usually indicated include severe hypertension, epilepsy, asthma, diabetes, heart disease, and infection. Drug therapy may be adjusted to minimize risks to both mother and fetus. Remember, if left untreated, these conditions endanger the fetus as well as the mother.

PLANNING TREATMENT FOR TWO
About 10 months ago, Marge Nelson, age 32, was diagnosed as having adult-onset diabetes. Since then, she's been successfully controlling her diabetes with tolbutamide (Orinase), 500 mg P.O. twice a day. About 1 week ago, Ms. Nelson learned that she's pregnant. Because Orinase increases the risk of fetal death (during the first trimester) and of neonatal hypoglycemia (when taken during the third trimester), Ms. Nelson's doctor discontinued Orinase therapy. Now she's taking a daily dose of insulin subcutaneously, titrated according to her serum glucose levels. Following her pregnancy, Ms. Nelson will probably return to Orinase or a similar oral hypoglycemic.

As Ms. Nelson's case illustrates, drug therapy in a pregnant patient must be closely correlated with the gestational age of the fetus. Whether a particular drug adversely affects the fetus depends on the stage of fetal growth and development at

CONTINUED ON PAGE 64

PREGNANCY

**PLANNING
TREATMENT FOR TWO
CONTINUED**

the time of drug exposure. The first and third trimesters warrant the most serious consideration, since the fetus is most vulnerable to drug effects at these times. But keep in mind that drug therapy may endanger the fetus at *any* point during the pregnancy.

Fetal risks: First trimester. During the first 3 weeks after conception, certain drugs may cause spontaneous abortion. From the 3rd to about the 10th week of gestation, fetal organ development begins. If certain drugs reach the fetus at this point, serious malformations may occur in the developing organs. High-risk drugs include alcohol, phenytoin, and metronidazole (Flagyl).

Fetal risks: Third trimester. During the third trimester, physiologic changes occur that allow more drug molecules to reach the fetus, thus increasing the risk of adverse reactions. These physiologic changes include:
• increased uteroplacental blood flow
• increased placental surface area
• decreased thickness of the semipermeable lipid membrane between placental capillaries and maternal blood vessels
• decreased maternal albumin levels, making more free drug available for placental transfer.

Because of these factors, the doctor will try to avoid giving a pregnant patient any drugs during the third trimester. For example, he'll avoid ordering sulfonamide antibiotics because these drugs can cause hyperbilirubinemia and kernicterus (bilirubin encephalopathy).

**OVER-THE-COUNTER PREPARATIONS:
SOME DO'S AND DON'TS FOR THE PREGNANT PATIENT**

Some over-the-counter (OTC) preparations, when taken in small doses and for short periods of time, can be safely used by the pregnant patient. But most preparations pose the same risks to the fetus as prescription drugs.

Urge your patient to play it safe by checking with her doctor or pharmacist before taking any medication. Keep a careful record of all drugs she's taking (including OTC products), and update it at each prenatal visit.

For information about the most commonly used OTC products and their implications in pregnancy, read what follows.

• **Aspirin.** Under certain circumstances, aspirin can be safe and effective for the pregnant patient. However, large doses taken over long periods of time can cause the following adverse reactions:
—prolonged gestation
—longer labor
—excessive maternal hemorrhage following delivery
—fetal or neonatal hemorrhage
—in utero closure of the ductus arteriosus.

• **Decongestants, antihistamines, antitussives.** When taken in large doses over long periods of time during pregnancy, these drugs can cause fetal addiction. Signs of withdrawal in the newborn include tremulousness, agitation, irritability, shrill crying, and poor feeding. If your pregnant patient requires a cold preparation, advise her to check with her doctor and to follow his orders exactly.

• **Vitamins.** Your pregnant patient should take vitamins only under doctor's orders. Large doses of

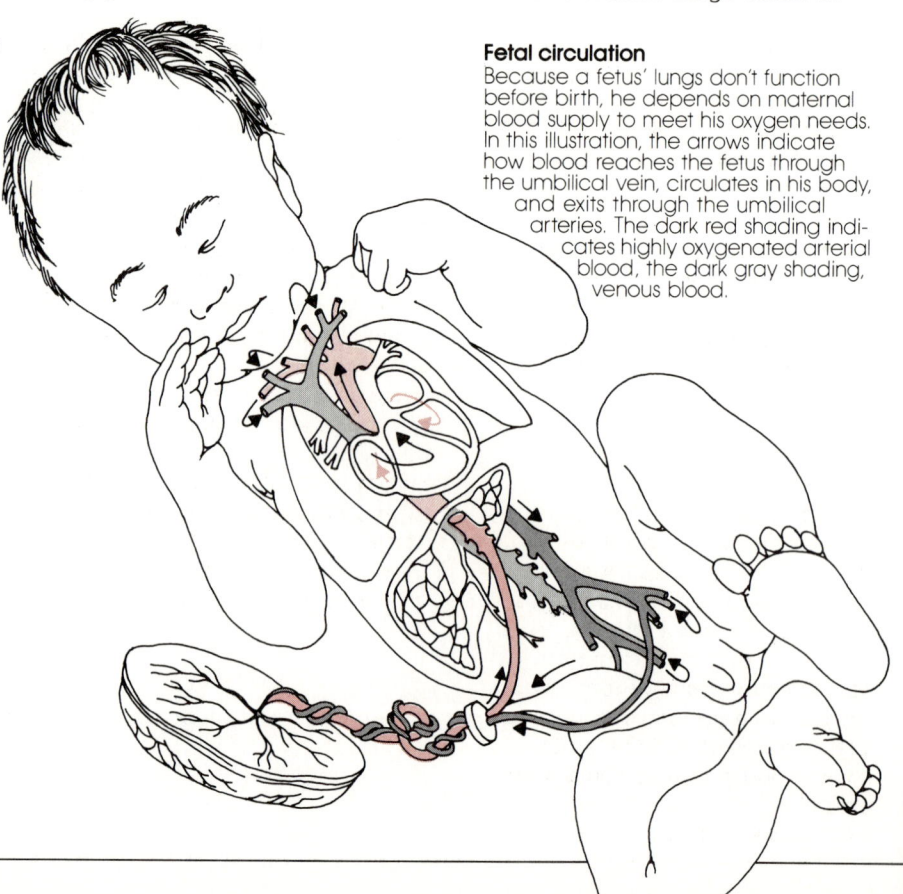

Fetal circulation
Because a fetus' lungs don't function before birth, he depends on maternal blood supply to meet his oxygen needs. In this illustration, the arrows indicate how blood reaches the fetus through the umbilical vein, circulates in his body, and exits through the umbilical arteries. The dark red shading indicates highly oxygenated arterial blood, the dark gray shading, venous blood.

64 MODIFYING DRUG THERAPY

vitamins A and D have been related to a wide range of congenital abnormalities. Also teach your patient that taking multiple vitamins doesn't compensate for poor nutrition.
• **Laxatives and stool softeners.** These preparations should be used only if dietary modifications fail to relieve the patient's constipation. Recommended bulk laxatives, such as Metamucil, include natural vegetable concentrates. Be sure to caution your patient about excessive cathartic use, which may induce labor.
• **Antidiarrheal preparations.** Kaopectate and similar preparations may be used in moderation.
• **Sedatives.** Excessive use of sedatives containing antihistamines can decrease fetal activity and cause fetal addiction. Withdrawal signs in the neonate include irritability, agitation, tremulousness, shrill crying, and poor feeding.
• **Caffeine.** Excessive consumption of coffee, tea, and various nondiet colas containing caffeine may produce restlessness and irritability in the fetus and newborn. Though the teratogenic effects of high caffeine consumption are unproven, advise your patient to avoid caffeine-containing stimulants, such as No Doz*, Vivarin*, and Caffedrine.
• **Artificial sweeteners.** The ability of such substances as saccharin, aspartame, and cyclamates (no longer marketed in the United States) to produce adverse fetal reactions is still under investigation. However, we do know that these substances readily cross the placenta. Advise your patient to use commercial preparations only in moderation. Some examples are Sweet 'N Low, NutraSweet, and products containing them.

*Not available in Canada

DRUG THERAPY FOR FETAL HEALTH PROBLEMS

In recent years, fetal health problems that are amenable to drug therapy have been successfully treated in utero. The treatment is still controversial. But when recommended, treatment is usually administered in one of two ways: the appropriate drug may be given to the mother for transfer to a specific fetal organ through the placenta; or the drug may be injected directly into the amniotic fluid, to be swallowed by the fetus. For a look at the most common fetal health problems that can be treated by in utero drug therapy, see the chart below.

DIAGNOSIS	CAUSE	DRUG THERAPY
Heart failure	Severe anemia	Digoxin
Hypothyroidism	Use of propylthiouracil by mother	Sodium levothyroxine
Biotin dependency	Genetic disorder	Biotin
Syphilis exposure	Maternal syphilis	Penicillin
Probable development of hyaline membrane disease following birth	Anticipated premature birth	Glucocorticoids

DRUGS AND THE NEONATE

Besides monitoring your patient's drug use during pregnancy, you must carefully monitor the neonate's reaction to drugs that crossed the placenta during labor and delivery. For example, analgesics and anesthetics depress the newborn's central nervous system. Large amounts of intravenous fluids may cause convulsions or an electrolyte imbalance. Excessive uterine stimulants may cause neonatal anoxic encephalopathy.

Fortunately, these adverse reactions are easily recognized and usually disappear as the neonate eliminates the drug from his system.

Keep in mind, however, that because the neonate's liver and kidneys are immature, drugs given to the mother during labor and delivery (as well as maternal hormones) may linger in his system for quite some time. This consideration is especially important to prevent possible adverse drug interactions if the neonate requires drug therapy for a particular health problem; for example, a congenital heart defect.

PREGNANCY

DRUGS AND BREAST-FEEDING

When a woman is breast-feeding, most drugs she takes appear in her breast milk. You can help protect the newborn from possible adverse reactions by counseling your patient about the implications of drug use while breast-feeding.

Considering risk factors. These factors influence the effects that drugs excreted in breast milk may have on a breast-fed infant:

• *Age of the newborn.* During the first week after delivery, drugs pass more easily from maternal blood plasma into colostrum, the substance initially secreted by a lactating woman. Also, during the first week certain drugs may compete with bilirubin for conjugation in the infant's liver. If bilirubin can't bind with protein and remains free in the infant's circulation, kernicterus may develop. (This risk is especially high for premature infants.)

In an infant who's 1 to 2 weeks old, the mechanisms of detoxification (acetylation, conjugation, and oxidation) aren't functioning fully. Together with an immature renal system, these factors place the newborn at high risk of accumulating toxic drug levels.

As the infant matures and becomes more capable of metabolizing drugs, his risk of adverse reactions from drugs in the mother's milk decreases.

• *Maternal health problems.* If the breast-feeding mother has renal disease or impairment, her kidneys excrete drugs more slowly than usual. As a result, drug concentration in breast milk may increase.

• *Method of drug administration.* Intravenously administered drugs reach higher concentrations in the mother's circulation than drugs given intramuscularly or orally.

• *Drug concentration.* Drug concentrations in breast milk are usually high when the mother's plasma drug levels are high—generally shortly after she takes a drug dose. Consequently, advise your patient to nurse the infant *before* taking her medication, *not after*.

> *Over-the-counter decongestants may diminish milk flow in a woman who is breast-feeding.*

• *Molecular weight.* Drugs with a molecular weight of less than 200 readily pass into breast milk, as do large, lipid-soluble, nonionized drug molecules.

• *Volume of ingested milk.* The amount of milk a newborn consumes at a particular feeding will influence the amount of drug that enters his system.

Protecting the infant. Some drugs, including those listed below, readily enter breast milk and adversely affect the infant. If your patient must take any of these drugs, tell her to discontinue breast-feeding throughout drug therapy.

—Antineoplastic drugs
—Oral anticoagulants
—Some anti-infectives, including chloramphenicol (Chloromycetin), nalidixic acid (NegGram), and tetracyclines
—Atropine
—Central nervous system (CNS) drugs, such as bromides and lithium
—Ergot alkaloids, such as methysergide maleate (Sansert)
—Estrogen (in high doses)
—Gold salts
—Indomethacin
—Radioactive substances.

Note: Your patient may safely take some anti-infective drugs while breast-feeding. Check with the doctor or pharmacist.

THE BREAST-FED INFANT: SPECIAL CONSIDERATIONS

In some circumstances, the doctor may order one of the following drugs for your patient—even though these drugs may cause adverse reactions in the breast-fed infant. To ensure the infant's safety, closely monitor his condition. Read what follows for the signs and symptoms you should watch for.

DRUG	POSSIBLE ADVERSE REACTIONS
Ampicillin	Rash, diarrhea, drug sensitivity, candidiasis
Analgesics	Lethargy, poor feeding, drowsiness
Anticonvulsants	Drowsiness
Cathartics	Gastrointestinal hypermotility
Isoniazid (INH)	Peripheral neuritis
Oral hypoglycemics	Hypoglycemia
Penicillin G	Drug sensitivity, candidiasis
Propranolol (Inderal)	Bradycardia
Psychotropics	Lethargy, poor feeding, drowsiness
Salicylates	Internal bleeding

66   MODIFYING DRUG THERAPY

PEDIATRICS

How Drugs Act in Children

In a child, a drug undergoes the same processes as in an adult: absorption, distribution, metabolism, and excretion. But while the basic steps are the same, a child's distinctive physiology changes some of the details. And this affects how he responds to drug therapy.

Before you administer drugs to your pediatric patient, make sure you understand the following age-related considerations. Use this information to reduce your patient's risk of adverse reactions and interactions while ensuring the effectiveness of drug therapy.

Absorption. The rate and completeness of drug absorption in the pediatric patient vary according to administration route. Keep these factors in mind.

Oral administration. Several physiologic differences reduce absorption of orally administered drugs in a child. These include:
• differences in the composition of intestinal flora
• slower GI tract motility
• underdeveloped transport mechanisms that carry drug particles across the intestinal membrane
• low gastric acidity.

Of all these factors, low gastric acidity is the most important. Until a child reaches age 3, his gastric fluids are less acidic than an adult's. This improves absorption of some drugs; for example, orally administered penicillin G. In an adult, gastric acid degrades the drug, causing poor or erratic absorption. But in an infant, whose gastric fluids are less acidic, penicillin G is better absorbed.

The child's activity level also affects GI absorption. During exercise, blood is shunted away from the GI tract to the arms and legs, decreasing GI blood supply and reducing drug absorption.

Topical administration. Unlike most drugs administered orally, topically administered drugs are absorbed faster and more completely in a child than in an adult. Absorption increases because the child's keratin and epithelial layers are much thinner than an adult's. In fact, some topically administered drugs can cause serious adverse reactions. Hydrocortisone ointment, for example, can suppress growth after long-term use. And antibiotic ointments, such as bacitracin, may trigger an allergy, especially if applied in excessive amounts.

> **SPECIAL NOTE:** Certain infant formulas and milk products increase gastric pH (*decrease* acidity) and interfere with absorption of acidic drugs. Give an infant oral medications between feedings, when his stomach is empty.

Intramuscular administration. Drugs administered intramuscularly are absorbed erratically in young children, especially newborns and infants. One reason is their relatively low muscle mass. In addition, blood flow to muscle tissue is variable, making absorption rates difficult to predict.

Distribution. As in an adult, drug distribution in a infant or child is influenced by plasma protein binding, body mass, and membrane permeability. Let's consider them one by one.

Protein binding. Because a child has fewer plasma proteins, he has fewer protein-binding sites than an adult. Moreover, endogenous substances, such as steroids and hormones, compete for those binding sites. As a result, more free (active) drug is available for receptor sites. Conditions such as malnutrition can further reduce the child's protein-binding capabilities by reducing the amount of plasma protein.

Body mass. A newborn or infant has a much higher percentage of body fluid and lower percentage of body fat than an older patient. Because of this, water-soluble drugs administered to an infant are distributed faster, while lipid-soluble drugs are distributed more slowly.

Keep this factor in mind when you treat a dehydrated child with a drug such as aspirin. Since he has less extracellular fluid for the drug to distribute into, normal doses can cause greater-than-usual plasma drug concentrations. As a result, he's at greater risk of toxicity.

Note: Body surface area correlates closely to a child's extracellular fluid volume. Because extracellular fluid volume is so important to drug distribution in an infant or child, pediatric drug dosages are commonly calculated on the basis of body surface area rather than body weight. (For details, see page 68.)

Membrane permeability. Because the child's blood-brain barrier is immature, certain drugs can penetrate to the central nervous system more easily. Lipid-soluble drugs, for example, readily cross the blood-brain barrier, possibly causing CNS toxicity.

Metabolism. Because an infant's liver is immature, his hepatic enzyme system isn't fully developed. Consequently, many drugs are metabolized slowly, increasing the risk of toxicity.

Gray baby syndrome, for example, results from a newborn's inability to metabolize chloramphenicol. If the doctor must order this drug for an infant under age

CONTINUED ON PAGE 68

MODIFYING DRUG THERAPY 67

PEDIATRICS

How Drugs Act in Children
CONTINUED

1 month, he'll reduce the usual pediatric dosage to 25 mg/kg/day and closely monitor plasma drug levels.

In a few cases, the child's age determines his ability to metabolize a drug. For example, a child between ages 6 months and 9 years metabolizes theophylline derivatives more quickly than patients who are either younger or older. To compensate for this rapid metabolism, a child in this age range needs a higher dosage (based on weight) than an adult.

Excretion. An infant's glomerular filtration rate reaches an adult level at about age 1; his tubular secretion rate reaches an adult level at about age 6 months. In the first month, a newborn's filtration rate may be as low as 5% of an adult's. Conditions such as kidney disease or dehydration decrease filtration. The doctor will consider these factors when determining drug dosage.

Calculating a Pediatric Dose

Let's say that the doctor's ordered 50 mg phenytoin (Dilantin Infatabs) P.O. for 7-year-old Steven Gorley. Before you give the drug, you're responsible for determining whether this dose is appropriate for him. Take the following steps.

First, weigh and measure the child. Then, find his height and weight measurements on the nomogram shown below, and connect these points with a straightedge. Next, look down the surface area scale to where the straightedge intersects the scale. That point indicates the child's surface area.

Now, use the *surface area rule* in the gray-shaded box below to determine the appropriate dose.

$$\frac{\text{adult dose} \times \text{surface area of child (in square meters)}}{1.7}$$

NOMOGRAM

Height cm | in	Surface Area m²	Weight lb | kg

Source: Behrman, Richard, and Vaughan, Victor, NELSON TEXTBOOK OF PEDIATRICS, 12th ed. Philadelphia: W.B. Saunders Co., 1983.

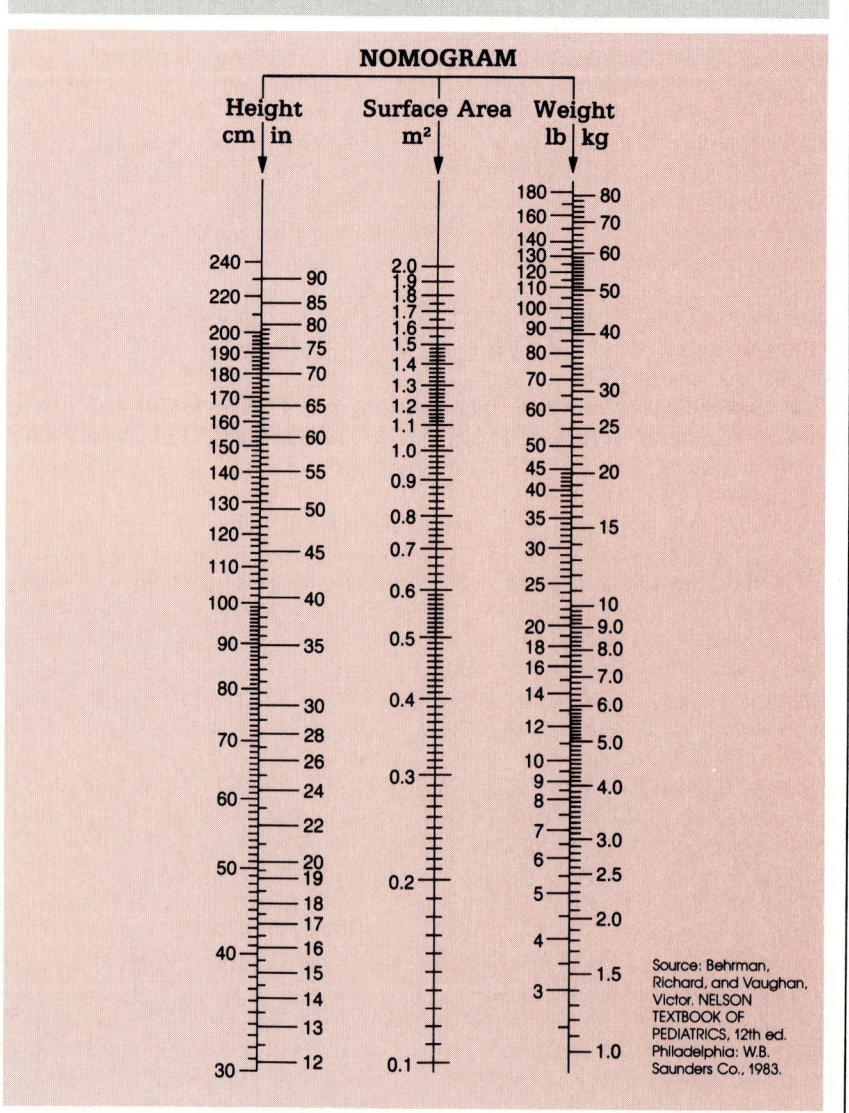

GERIATRICS

THE ELDERLY: SPECIAL PATIENTS WITH SPECIAL NEEDS

Nowadays, people are living longer and fuller lives than ever before. Consequently, you're probably caring for more and more people over age 60. Chances are, you're also giving them more drugs and seeing more serious adverse reactions and interactions than with younger patients.

Why are the elderly so susceptible to adverse reactions? And why are these reactions so much more serious than in younger patients? For answers, you must consider several factors.

To begin with, the aging process produces physiologic changes that can significantly alter drug actions and effects, possibly causing an adverse reaction. If such a reaction occurs, many of the same physiologic changes that contributed to the reaction also limit the patient's ability to cope with it. As a result, an adverse reaction may have more serious consequences for an elderly patient than it would for someone younger.

Further complicating the picture is the fact that many elderly patients develop chronic illnesses requiring drug therapy. Most of these patients take several different prescription medications daily; they may regularly use over-the-counter drugs as well. Each time a patient adds a new drug to his daily regimen, regardless of whether it's prescribed, he increases his risk of experiencing adverse drug reactions and interactions.

Your patient may need several drugs to maintain his health and enjoy his accustomed life-style. You can help him minimize the special risks he faces by following the guidelines in the next few pages.

DRUG ACTION IN THE ELDERLY PATIENT

The aging process changes an elderly patient's anatomy and physiology in ways that alter many body functions. Though age-related changes aren't always apparent, they can significantly alter drug action. Here's how.

Absorption. Although some studies indicate that drug absorption from the GI tract is unaffected by the aging process, other studies suggest that aging reduces the absorption rate in an elderly patient for several reasons. First, decreased hydrochloric acid secretion may reduce the acidity of stomach contents. As a result, oral drugs that require an acid medium for absorption are either absorbed more slowly or not at all. These drugs include iron, salicylates, oral anticoagulants, nitrofurantoin (Furadantin), probenecid (Benemid), digoxin, and tetracycline (Achromycin, Tetracyn).

Second, intestinal villi become shorter and broader with age, decreasing the intestine's surface area. Finally, reduced GI motility and blood flow may also decrease absorption.

Distribution. Drug distribution in an elderly patient slows for several reasons. First, his plasma protein levels (particularly his albumin levels) decrease, reducing the number of protein-binding sites. As a result, the amount of free drug increases, and the drug remains active in the patient's system longer.

In addition, a patient's active and passive transport systems function less efficiently as he ages. This impedes drug transfer across tissue membranes.

Changes in the elderly patient's body mass also affect drug distribution. With age, water volume and lean tissue diminish. Since water-soluble drugs normally distribute to body fluid and lean tissue, the reduced availability of either increases the concentration of these drugs in their free (active) forms. Conversely, because the proportion of fatty tissue increases with age, the body retains lipid-soluble drugs for longer periods of time, which prolongs their action.

Metabolism. Decreased hepatic blood flow, smaller liver size, and reduced production of enzymes that break down most drugs slow drug metabolism in the elderly

---

Because the elderly are prone to chronic diseases—especially those affecting kidney, liver, and cardiovascular function—they're predisposed to adverse drug reactions and interactions.

---

patient. As a result, drugs remain active in his system longer. These metabolic changes can be further aggravated by medical conditions, such as congestive heart failure.

Excretion. The kidneys are the primary excretion site for most drugs (or their metabolites), including such commonly ordered drugs as digoxin, most antibiotics, hypoglycemic agents, and diuretics. But because renal blood flow diminishes during the aging process, the elderly patient's kidneys filter and excrete these drugs more slowly. And because fewer of his renal tubules continue to function, glomerular filtration, tubular reabsorption, and active tubular secretion progress more slowly.

The combined effect of these age-related changes is a longer

CONTINUED ON PAGE 70

MODIFYING DRUG THERAPY 69

GERIATRICS

DRUG ACTION IN THE ELDERLY PATIENT CONTINUED

half-life for most drugs, a factor that can cause drug toxicity in the elderly patient. To prevent such an occurrence, carefully monitor your elderly patient's kidney function and his response to drug therapy. Reevaluate therapy whenever a drug is added or deleted from the regimen; as ordered, modify therapy appropriately.

As a patient ages, tissue sensitivity changes, heightening the effects of some drugs. As a result, more of these drugs remain active in the patient's system. This is especially true of barbiturates, which are especially potent for elderly patients.

Decreased hormonal secretion may affect drug action at receptor sites. Replacement therapy may be necessary to counteract the decline. Once therapy begins, you must carefully monitor the patient for enhanced drug response, since replacement therapy can increase the sensitivity of receptor sites.

Finally, keep in mind that aging can affect a patient's compliance as well as his physiologic response to drug therapy. Cerebral arteriosclerosis, for example, can cause many behavioral disorders, including memory loss, confusion, and lethargy. These problems, in turn, can lead to poor compliance, accidental overdose, or use of the wrong drug.

But don't make the mistake of assuming that a patient exhibiting behavioral disorders associated with old age is senile. He may be experiencing adverse reactions from one or more of his drugs. If so, you can take steps to help him. For guidelines on distinguishing between senility and adverse drug reactions, see page 72.

ENHANCING PATIENT COMPLIANCE

A common cause of adverse drug reactions is poor compliance with the prescribed drug regimen. Helping your patient to follow his drug regimen exactly is an essential part of the drug therapy program you develop for him.

Assuring your patient's compliance while he's hospitalized is fairly easy since you administer his medication and carefully monitor his reactions. But once he's discharged, his compliance with the prescribed drug regimen may diminish. He may fail to take the prescribed doses, take inappropriate doses, forget to take his medication at the appropriate times, prematurely discontinue his medication, or take medications prescribed for previous disorders.

Such noncompliance, usually unintentional, can be caused by a number of age-related changes that decrease the elderly patient's perception, recall, and motor skills. In addition, he may be living on a fixed income, limiting his ability to pay for medication. Familiarizing yourself with these possible problems will help you take appropriate measures to improve compliance. Keep the following points in mind.

Hearing. Hearing loss can prevent the elderly patient from hearing instructions completely and correctly. As a result, he may take a drug dose at the wrong time or in the wrong way. For example, he may swallow a drug that he should have chewed or put under his tongue.

Vision. Loss of visual acuity and the ability to discriminate colors, as well as glare from eyeglasses, can interfere with the patient's ability to comply. Vision problems limit his ability to read instructions, differentiate among pills and capsules, or spot drug deterioration.

Note: Patients see reds and yellows best, blues and greens the worst.

Muscle strength and coordination. Decreased muscle strength and coordination, as well as arthritic joints, can make removing bottle caps (especially childproof caps) difficult or impossible.

Finances. If your elderly patient is on a fixed income, he may try to make his medications last longer by skipping doses or prolonging dosage intervals. And he may fail to refill prescriptions that he needs.

To help your patient overcome these age-related drawbacks and improve his compliance with his drug regimen, consider the following tips:

• *Hearing your instructions.* To make sure your patient hears and understands his dosage instructions, eliminate background noise during teaching sessions. Speak slowly and distinctly while facing him. Make your instructions as specific as possible.

Keep in mind that your patient may be embarrassed to admit that he can't hear well. To make sure he understands you, ask him to repeat the instructions you give him. Writing down the instructions may help, too.

• *Reading medication labels.* If your patient's medication is packaged in an amber container, tape the label on the outside so it won't be obscured by the tinted glass. Or ask the pharmacist to package the patient's medication in clear bottles (unless contraindicated). This may help your patient identify his medication by appearance.

You can also print the dosage instructions and schedule on a separate sheet of paper, using large letters, and tape a small tablet or capsule to the schedule. Then your patient, his family,

MODIFYING DRUG THERAPY

or a visiting nurse can easily refer to them.
- *Opening medication bottles.* If your patient has arthritis or Parkinson's disease, tell him to ask the pharmacist for standard bottle caps whenever he gets his prescriptions refilled. (Remind him to keep his medications out of children's reach.)
- *Using social service resources.* If your patient has a limited income, refer him to a social service representative for information on financial aid, and ask the doctor to prescribe generic drugs. Also inquire about the patient's eating habits—an elderly patient may habitually skip meals in an effort to save money. If so, he may miss medication doses scheduled with meals.

Work together with him to plan a realistic schedule (or ask the dietitian to help him). If necessary, contact a social service program, such as Meals on Wheels, to help him begin eating properly.

GERIATRIC DRUG USE: A CLOSER LOOK

According to a recent survey by the National Center for Health Statistics, the drug types shown in this pie graph were most often ordered for geriatric patients. The figures given for each slice of the pie indicate the percentage distribution for each drug.

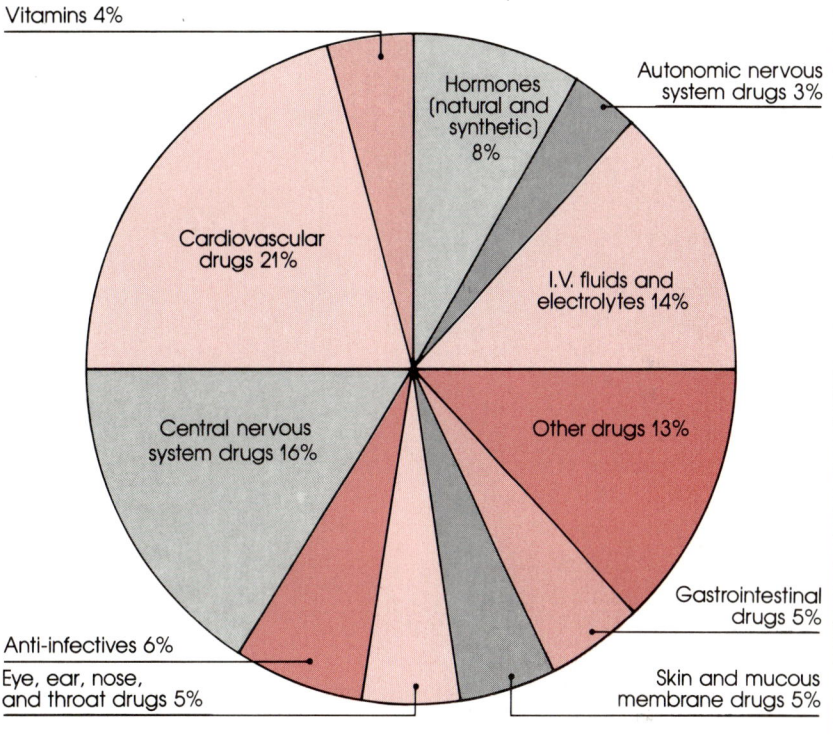

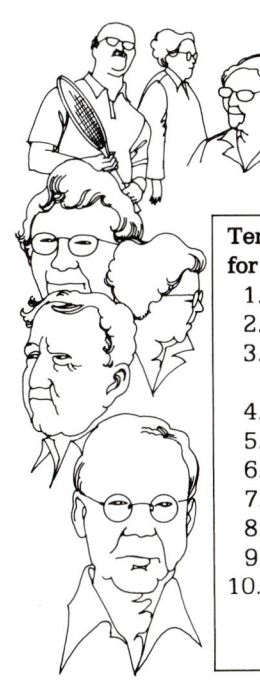

- Vitamins 4%
- Hormones (natural and synthetic) 8%
- Autonomic nervous system drugs 3%
- Cardiovascular drugs 21%
- I.V. fluids and electrolytes 14%
- Central nervous system drugs 16%
- Other drugs 13%
- Anti-infectives 6%
- Eye, ear, nose, and throat drugs 5%
- Gastrointestinal drugs 5%
- Skin and mucous membrane drugs 5%

Ten most commonly ordered drugs for females ages 65 and older
1. Digoxin (Lanoxin)
2. Furosemide (Lasix)
3. Triamterene and hydrochlorothiazide (Dyazide)
4. Propranolol (Inderal)
5. Methyldopa (Aldomet)
6. Vitamin B_{12}
7. Digoxin (all brands)
8. Ibuprofen (Motrin)
9. Insulin
10. Hydrochlorothiazide (all brands)

Ten most commonly ordered drugs for males ages 65 and older
1. Furosemide (Lasix)
2. Digoxin (Lanoxin)
3. Propranolol (Inderal)
4. Digoxin (all brands)
5. Isosorbide (Isordil)
6. Triamterene and hydrochlorothiazide (Dyazide)
7. Aspirin
8. Hydrochlorothiazide (all brands)
9. Hydrochlorothiazide (HydroDIURIL)
10. Prednisone

Source: National Center for Health Statistics

MODIFYING DRUG THERAPY

GERIATRICS

SENILITY OR ADVERSE REACTIONS?

"I've been so forgetful lately," says Mr. Hopkins, your 73-year-old patient. "But I guess I should expect that at my age."

Like your patient, you may mistakenly assume that confusion, forgetfulness, and other symptoms associated with senility are almost inevitable for an elderly patient. But don't overlook another possibility. If Mr. Hopkins is undergoing drug therapy, he may be experiencing an adverse drug reaction or interaction. With appropriate modification of therapy, the doctor may be able to correct or minimize your patient's symptoms.

What can you do? Review the following guidelines. Then read the chart below for more details about drugs that can cause symptoms often attributed to aging.

• Help the doctor determine the lowest effective dose by monitoring your patient for therapeutic effects and adverse reactions until steady-state blood concentrations have been attained. Document your observations.

• To help your patient remember his medications, write down the name and dosage of each and the reason for taking it. Tell him to keep this list with his pill containers.

• Teach your patient to watch for possible adverse reactions to drug therapy. Tell him which reactions to report immediately.

• Warn him against using anyone else's medication (or giving his to anyone else).

• Review his drug regimen. Be alert for drugs (or drug combinations) that may cause symptoms resembling senility. If you suspect that your patient's reaction is drug-related, alert the doctor so he can adjust drug therapy.

SYMPTOMS	POSSIBLE CAUSES
Confusion	Methyldopa, digoxin, and cimetidine
Depression	Reserpine
Anorexia	Digoxin
Weakness	Certain diuretics, such as furosemide and hydrochlorothiazide, which can deplete potassium
Lethargy and drowsiness	Various antianxiety agents, analgesics, antihistamines, and sleep medications, including chlorpromazine and pentobarbital
Ataxia	Phenytoin, very high doses of flurazepam (and other sedatives), or hypnotics
Forgetfulness	Barbiturates and methyldopa
Constipation	Medications with anticholinergic properties, such as belladonna-containing drugs, narcotics, tricyclic antidepressants, and iron preparations
Diarrhea	Antacid preparations containing magnesium; quinidine

GENETICS

DRUGS AND GENETIC DISPOSITION

In addition to age and a condition such as pregnancy, genetic makeup can alter your patient's response to drug therapy. Pharmacogenetics, the study of the relationship between drugs and genetic makeup, explores how genetic disorders can produce adverse and idiosyncratic reactions to certain drugs. By keeping genetic factors in mind, you can significantly minimize adverse reactions in patients with genetic disorders. Depending on your patient's condition, you may do this by modifying drug dosage or avoiding drugs that are known to cause adverse reactions in patients who have the disorder.

Many individuals, because of a hereditary defect, either lack an enzyme necessary to detoxify certain drugs or have insufficient amounts of it. In some patients, the abnormality significantly alters drug response. In others, abnormal enzyme activity can cause physical or biochemical changes that affect several organ systems. Tests are available to detect only a few of the known genetic deficiencies. But additional tests are being developed. In the future, genetic profiles may become as routine as a patient's laboratory workup and may provide as much information.

For the time being, however, you'll have to rely on your knowledge of the various types of genetic disorders and the adverse reactions associated with them. The information that follows will help.

G6PD DEFICIENCY: A CASE IN POINT

Several months ago, Claire Prete, a 54-year-old legal assistant, burned her left leg in a car accident. About a week ago, she arrived on your unit following reconstructive surgery on her leg. She was feeling fine until a few days ago, when she began to complain of frequent and painful urination. Because a culture and urinalysis indicated a urinary tract infection, her doctor prescribed sulfisoxazole (Gantrisin), 1 g, P.O. four times a day.

About 3 days after she began Gantrisin therapy, Ms. Prete complained of weakness, chills, and abdominal pain; in addition, her urine became unusually dark. What's wrong with your patient?

Based on these signs and symptoms, you might think that Ms. Prete's urinary tract infection had worsened. But the results of a urinalysis and complete blood cell count indicate that Ms. Prete has hemolytic anemia. The source of her problem is actually a genetic deficiency that's altered the action of Gantrisin.

Ms. Prete is deficient in an enzyme called glucose-6-phosphate dehydrogenase (G6PD). Normally, G6PD helps protect red blood cells from destruction by drugs such as Gantrisin. But in patients like Ms. Prete, such drugs destroy red blood cells. The result: Hemolytic anemia.

Patients most likely to develop hemolytic anemia as a result of a G6PD deficiency are people of Mediterranean descent and blacks. In blacks, the anemia is usually mild and self-limiting. But for other people deficient in G6PD, hemolytic anemia can be severe. For these patients, Gantrisin should be substituted with another drug that's not known to produce this reaction.

G6PD hemolysis
This illustration of a blood smear shows the hemolysis that occurs in G6PD deficiency. As you see, some of the red blood cells have a fragmented, or bitten, appearance.

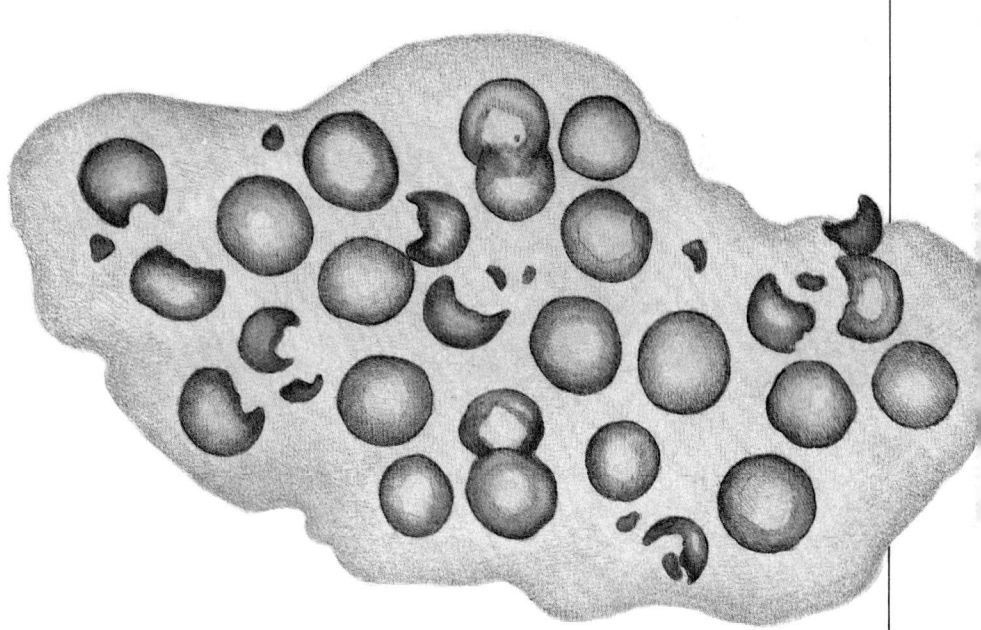

TAKING PRECAUTIONS

Can you prevent an adverse reaction from a genetic deficiency like G6PD? Probably not. Why? Because, like your patient, you'll probably be unaware that a genetic deficiency exists until a telltale adverse reaction occurs. You can, however, take some precautions by following these guidelines:
• Obtain a thorough patient history. Since many genetic disorders occur more frequently among certain races and nationalities, be sure to ask the patient about genetic history, including ethnic background.
• Ask the patient if he or any family members are sensitive to specific drugs. If the answer's *yes*, question him further to identify the nature of the reaction. Remember, a patient with a genetic deficiency may mistakenly assume that his symptoms are caused by an allergy.
• If you know that your patient has a genetic deficiency, familiarize yourself with the drugs that may be affected by it. For details, see the chart on pages 74 and 75.
• Carefully monitor your patient's condition while he's on drug therapy. Inform the doctor at the first sign or symptom of an adverse reaction.
• Be sure your patient knows what drug he's taking, why he's taking it, how and when he should take it, and what adverse reactions he may experience.
• If your patient has a history of genetically induced drug reactions, recommend that he wear a Medic Alert bracelet or necklace identifying his condition and the drugs he's sensitive to.

GENETICS

RECOGNIZING PHARMACOGENETIC REACTIONS

Because genetic deficiencies are relatively rare, you've probably cared for very few patients with pharmacogenetic disorders. But if you do care for such a patient, you must be prepared to protect him from adverse reactions by familiarizing yourself with his condition and the drugs that may trigger an adverse reaction. To do so, use the following chart as a guide.

GENETIC CONDITION	PATIENT POPULATION	DRUGS CAUSING ADVERSE REACTIONS	POSSIBLE ADVERSE REACTIONS
Glucose-6-phosphate dehydrogenase (G6PD) deficiency, an enzyme deficiency found in more than 80 forms that leads to red blood cell destruction by certain drugs	*In its severe form* (Mediterranean variant): Greeks, Sardinians, Sephardic Jews, and Asian and Northwest Indians *In its less severe form:* Blacks and southern Chinese. *Note:* More males than females are affected.	• Antimalarials, such as primaquine and quinacrine (Atabrine*) • Sulfonamides and sulfones, such as sulfamethoxazole (one of the drugs in Bactrim and Septra), sulfasalazine (Azulfidine*), sulfisoxazole (Gantrisin), and sulfoxone • Urinary tract antiseptics and non-sulfonamide antibacterial agents, such as furazolidone (Furoxone*) and nitrofurantoin (Furadantin*) • Analgesics, such as aspirin and phenacetin • Chloramphenicol (Chloromycetin), in the Mediterranean variant • Quinine and quinidine, in the Mediterranean variant • Miscellaneous drugs, including diazoxide, dimercaprol, nalidixic acid (NegGram), penicillamine, vitamin K, and ascorbic acid (vitamin C) in large doses	• Mild to severe hemolysis, causing dark urine (from free hemoglobin), jaundice, weakness, and abdominal and back pain. If hemolysis is severe, the doctor will stop the drug. *Note:* Because hemolysis is usually mild and self-limiting in blacks, drug therapy may continue. However, increasing drug dosage may cause hemolysis to recur.
Slow acetylator, a condition caused by decreased liver enzyme activity, which reduces the rate at which the liver metabolizes various drugs	About 50% of American blacks and whites, 20% of American Indians, 13% of Japanese, and 5% of Eskimos	• Isoniazid (INH) • Hydralazine (Apresoline) • Procainamide (Pronestyl) • Dapsone (Avlosulfon) • Phenelzine (Nardil)	• Systemic lupus erythematosus-like syndrome with prolonged administration of INH, procainamide, and hydralazine • Peripheral neuritis and liver toxicity with INH • Changes in behavior and coordination with phenytoin
Atypical pseudocholinesterase	Europeans and Eskimos	• Succinylcholine (Anectine)	• Increased skeletal muscle relaxation and prolonged respiratory paralysis from potentiation of neuromuscular blockade

*Not available in Canada

74 MODIFYING DRUG THERAPY

GENETIC CONDITION	PATIENT POPULATION	DRUGS CAUSING ADVERSE REACTIONS	POSSIBLE ADVERSE REACTIONS
Warfarin resistance	Variable	• Warfarin sodium (Coumadin)	• Decreased response to warfarin • Increased vitamin K sensitivity, increasing clotting *Important:* Closely monitor the patient's prothrombin time throughout therapy.
Hepatic porphyria (three forms), characterized by excessive porphyrin production in the liver	*Acute intermittent porphyria:* Females, ages 15 to 40 *Porphyria cutanea tarda:* South African whites, ages 30 to 50	• Barbiturates, such as amobarbital (Amytal), pentobarbital (Nembutal), and secobarbital (Seconal) • Possibly sulfa drugs and chloroquine phosphate (Aralen Phosphate) • Miscellaneous drugs, such as phenytoin, methsuximide, methyldopa, chloramphenicol, and ergot preparations	• Photosensitivity, acute abdominal pain, neuropathy, and other signs and symptoms of porphyria
Malignant hyperthermia, a condition characterized by rapid temperature elevation ranging from 102.2° to 107.6° F. (39° to 42° C.), general muscle rigidity, and severe metabolic acidosis	Variable; symptoms appear in about 1 out of every 20,000 anesthetized patients, especially those premedicated with succinylcholine	• Potent inhalation anesthetics, such as nitrous oxide, methoxyflurane, halothane, ether, cyclopropane, or any of these drugs in combination; and, possibly, lidocaine and mepivacaine	• Damage to the brain and other vital organs, possibly leading to death *Note:* To treat the condition, give dantrolene sodium (Dantrium) I.V., as ordered.
Closed-angle glaucoma (increased intraocular pressure from obstruction of aqueous humor outflow)	About 1 in 4,000 whites	• Scopolamine • Mydriatics, such as atropine sulfate, phenylephrine hydrochloride (Neo-Synephrine) • Drugs with atropine-like anticholinergic effects, such as antihistamines, phenothiazines, and tricyclic antidepressants	• Angle closure in patients over age 30 • Exacerbation of glaucoma possible, resulting in permanent vision changes

MODIFYING DRUG THERAPY   75

KIDNEY DISEASE

DRUGS AND KIDNEY DISEASE

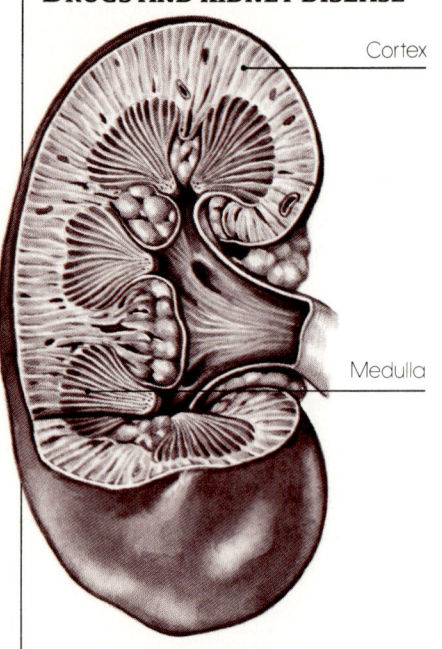

Renal failure: Gross anatomic changes
The kidney's thick cortex and darkened medulla, shown here, characterize acute renal failure. Possible causes include acute glomerular nephritis and toxic nephropathy.

Planning drug therapy for a patient with kidney disease isn't easy. Any impairment of kidney function affects the excretory rate of most drugs as well as their intensity and duration of action.

Many commonly prescribed drugs (especially antibiotics) and their active metabolites are excreted almost entirely by the kidneys. Impaired kidney function reduces drug excretion, possibly leading to drug accumulation.

If the patient's kidney function has been significantly diminished by injury, disease, or age, the doctor must consider ways to avoid or minimize toxicity and other adverse effects. Of course, avoiding drug therapy altogether is one answer. But this solution isn't always possible. If the patient needs drug therapy for multiple health problems, the doctor must plan a drug regimen that will minimize risks. To learn about your role, read the next few pages.

DRUGS REQUIRING RENAL EXCRETION: SOME EXAMPLES

The following commonly prescribed drugs (or their metabolites) are excreted primarily by the kidneys. If your patient has renal disease, make a dosage adjustment, as ordered.

ANTIBIOTICS
- Amikacin
- Ampicillin
- Carbenicillin
- Cefazolin
- Cephalothin
- Cloxacillin
- Gentamicin
- Kanamycin
- Methicillin
- Netilmicin
- Oxacillin
- Penicillin
- Streptomycin
- Tetracycline
- Ticarcillin
- Tobramycin

OTHER DRUGS
- Chlorpropamide
- Cimetidine
- Digoxin
- Disopyramide
- Meperidine
- Procainamide

ASSESSING KIDNEY FUNCTION

In patients with normal kidney function, drugs are filtered by the glomeruli and are then excreted, either unchanged or as active metabolites. (For details on normal kidney excretion, see pages 26 and 27.)

In patients with impaired kidney function, however, the glomerular filtration rate falls, and drugs are excreted slowly or not at all. As a result, drugs or their metabolites continue to circulate.

If a patient with impaired kidney function receives additional doses, drug concentration may reach toxic levels. As a result, the doctor will probably reduce the patient's drug dosage.

To determine appropriate dosage, the doctor may order the following tests.

• **Blood urea nitrogen and creatinine levels.** These tests help him assess your patient's renal function. (Creatinine levels are the more reliable indicator.)
• **24-hour urine test for creatinine clearance.** From test results, the doctor can estimate glomerular filtration rate. Once the doctor knows creatinine clearance, he can determine appropriate dosage using a special nomogram.
• **Protein testing.** This test can reveal the presence of protein in urine, which suggests renal dysfunction.

Note: A complete renal workup also includes renal computerized tomography, intravenous pyelogram, and renal angiography.

In addition, the doctor assesses the overall status of your patient's health and considers such variables as altered drug absorption, protein binding, and liver function. Of course, he'll also consider the potential effect of other medications the patient's taking.

Once the doctor establishes the patient's baseline renal function, he'll modify dosage accordingly. Chances are, he'll do one of the following:
• prescribe the same drug dose at extended intervals
• prescribe a reduced dose at the usual intervals.

Before you give your renal patient any medication, check the order carefully. If the dosage seems inappropriate, ask the doctor about it.

76 MODIFYING DRUG THERAPY

MONITORING DRUG THERAPY

Once your patient's begun drug therapy, carefully monitor his response. Keep the following important points in mind:
• Give the following drugs to a patient with a renal disease only with caution:
—tetracycline
—aspirin
—potassium-containing drugs like potassium penicillin
—products containing magnesium; for example, some antacids and milk of magnesia.

Also warn the patient not to use salt substitutes, which are high in potassium.
• Diseased kidneys are highly susceptible to drugs' nephrotoxic effects. Use these drugs only when absolutely necessary and with extreme caution. For examples of nephrotoxic drugs, see page 79.
• Your patient may be receiving diuretics to improve his kidney function. Use extreme caution when administering other drugs, since they may interact adversely with the diuretic. For example, furosemide, a loop diuretic, can potentiate the ototoxicity of all aminoglycoside antibiotics.
• If your patient is elderly, remember that serum creatinine levels may appear normal, despite impaired kidney function, because of decreased creatinine production. To accurately assess his renal function, closely monitor his urine output, creatinine clearance, urine electrolytes, the presence of protein in urine, and other urine test values.
• Help the doctor determine effective dosage for your patient. Throughout drug therapy, use plasma drug concentrations whenever possible, to assess the need for a dosage adjustment. If plasma concentrations aren't available for your patient's prescribed drugs, monitor his response and consult with the pharmacist or doctor.
• Caution your patient about the risks of using over-the-counter drugs. Advise him to check with the doctor or pharmacist before taking any such preparations.

DRUGS AND DIALYSIS

A patient with renal failure may also have other medical problems; for example, hypertension and congestive heart failure. Consequently, he may need a daily regimen of several different drugs, including vitamins.

If the patient is undergoing dialysis, ensuring safe and effective drug therapy is more difficult than usual. Dialysis removes some drugs and not others. Either way, drug therapy becomes complicated. If the drug is dialyzed, the patient may never experience its intended therapeutic effects. But if the drug *isn't* dialyzed, it may accumulate in his bloodstream and cause toxicity.

To protect your patient against either occurrence, first determine whether the drug (or drugs) he's taking is dialyzable (see page 78 for guidelines). If it is, consult with the doctor about dosage timing; he may want you to administer the drug after dialysis. (Never change dosage timing without the doctor's approval.)

If the drug isn't significantly dialyzable, expect the doctor to order a lower-than-usual dosage. If he doesn't, question him (or the pharmacist) before giving the drug. For details on how dialysis affects the drugs most commonly ordered for renal patients, read what follows.
• *Multivitamins*. Water-soluble vitamins, normally supplied by diet, are lost through dialysis. To replace them, the doctor may order daily doses of multivitamins and folic acid. Give these drugs *after* dialysis treatment.
• *Antacids and cathartics*. Preparations such as Maalox Plus, milk of magnesia, Mylanta, and magnesium citrate are contraindicated in dialysis patients. These products contain magnesium, which isn't readily eliminated by dialysis. Magnesium accumulation could cause toxicity.
• *Digitalis*. If your dialysis patient also has congestive heart failure, he may be taking digitalis, which isn't eliminated by dialysis. If the patient's taking digoxin, for example, the doctor may prescribe a dosage as low as 0.125 mg P.O., every other day or even every third day.
• *Antibiotics*. Your dialysis patient is highly susceptible to infection. If an infection develops, the doctor may order an antibiotic, such as gentamicin. As ordered, administer such an antibiotic at extended intervals or after dialysis.
• *Antihypertensives*. Many dialysis patients are hypertensive. For most, the condition is effectively controlled by such drugs as methyldopa, captopril, propranolol, prazosin, hydralazine, minoxidil, or clonidine. Since dialysis treatment normally lowers a patient's blood pressure, the doctor may order you to hold the antihypertensive drug dose that immediately precedes dialysis treatment.

KIDNEY DISEASE

Dialyzable drugs: some examples

Are the drugs your patient's taking dialyzable? Use the following chart as a quick reference, with this caution: It provides general guidelines only. The amount of drug removed by dialysis may vary from patient to patient, depending on such factors as:
- the patient's condition
- drug characteristics (for example, whether the drug has active metabolites)
- the duration of dialysis
- the dialysate used
- the rate of blood flow through the dialysis machine (in the case of hemodialysis) or the dialysate dwell time (in the case of peritoneal dialysis)
- the purpose of the procedure (for example, is the patient undergoing short-term dialysis treatment for drug overdose or long-term treatments for end-stage renal disease?)

What are the implications for your patient? Clearly, you can't safely make broad assumptions about the effects of dialysis on drug therapy. Don't assume that your patient needs an extra drug dose just because the drug is considered dialyzable. His individual response to treatment may make a dosage adjustment unnecessary. Consult the doctor.

DRUG	HEMODIALYSIS	PERITONEAL DIALYSIS
Analgesics		
acetaminophen	●	○
aspirin	●	●
methadone	○	○
propoxyphene	○	○
Antianxiety agents		
chlordiazepoxide	○	○
diazepam	○	○
meprobamate	●	●
Antiarrhythmics		
lidocaine	○	○
procainamide	●	X
propranolol	○	○
quinidine	●	●
Antidepressants		
amitriptyline	○	○
imipramine	○	○
nortriptyline	○	○
Antihypertensives		
clonidine	○	X
diazoxide	●	●
hydralazine	○	○
methyldopa	●	●
nitroprusside	●	●
reserpine	○	○
Anti-infectives		
amikacin	●	●
aminosalicylic acid	●	X
amoxicillin	●	X
amphotericin B	○	○
ampicillin	●	○
azlocillin	●	X
carbenicillin	●	○

DRUG	HEMODIALYSIS	PERITONEAL DIALYSIS
cefamandole	●	X
cefazolin	●	X
cephalexin	●	●
cephalothin	●	●
cephapirin	●	●
cephradine	●	●
chloramphenicol	●	○
chloroquine	○	○
clindamycin	○	○
cloxacillin	○	○
colistimethate	○	●
co-trimoxazole	●	○
dicloxacillin	○	○
doxycycline	○	○
erythromycin	○	○
ethambutol	●	●
flucytosine	●	●
gentamicin	●	●
isoniazid	●	●
kanamycin	●	●
lincomycin	○	○
methenamine mandelate	X	○
methicillin	○	○
metronidazole	●	X
minocycline	○	○
nafcillin	○	○
neomycin	●	X
nitrofurantoin	●	X
oxacillin	○	○
penicillin G	●	○
quinine	●	○
rifampin	○	○

DRUG	HEMODIALYSIS	PERITONEAL DIALYSIS
streptomycin	●	●
sulfamethoxazole	●	○
sulfisoxazole	●	●
tetracycline	○	○
ticarcillin	●	○
tobramycin	●	●
trimethoprim	●	○
vancomycin	○	○
Antineoplastics		
azathioprine	●	X
cyclophosphamide	●	X
5-fluorouracil	●	X
Digitalis glycosides		
digitoxin	○	○
digoxin	○	○
Sedatives and hypnotics		
ethchlorvynol	●	○
flurazepam	○	○
glutethimide	●	○
pentobarbital	○	○
phenobarbital	●	●
secobarbital	○	○
Miscellaneous		
chlorpromazine	○	○
folic acid	●	●
furosemide	○	○
heparin	○	○
lithium carbonate	●	●
phenytoin	○	○
theophylline	●	●
vitamins (water-soluble)	●	●

Key: ● Dialyzable   ○ Not dialyzable   X Insufficient or conflicting data

LIVER DISEASE

NEPHROTOXIC DRUGS

Even healthy kidneys can suffer functional damage from nephrotoxic drugs. If the kidneys are diseased, the risk increases.

As a class, antibiotics have the greatest potential for causing kidney damage. Read the list below for examples of antibiotics and other drugs recognized as nephrotoxic.

- Aminoglycosides
- Amphotericin B
- Captopril
- Cisplatin
- Cyclophosphamide
- Gold salts
- Indomethacin
- Lithium
- Mercurial diuretics
- Methicillin sodium
- Methotrexate
- Methoxyflurane
- Penicillamine
- Rifampin
- Polymyxin B
- Phenazopyridine
- Sulfonamides
- Tetracycline hydrochloride
- Vancomycin hydrochloride

Fortunately, most drug-caused nephrotoxicity is reversible. Depending on the amount of healthy tissue the kidney has in reserve, the kidney may begin to repair itself after the drug is discontinued. As renal function improves, dosages of other drugs may need adjustment.

DRUGS AND LIVER DISEASE

The impact of liver dysfunction on drug therapy varies from patient to patient. One of the body's most durable organs, the liver may continue to metabolize drugs despite severe parenchymal damage from such disorders as hepatitis or cirrhosis. But because normal liver function is impaired, drug metabolism is haphazard and unpredictable.

Assessment variables. How can you weigh the impact of liver disease on your patient's condition? Unfortunately, no single diagnostic test specifically and accurately quantifies either liver function or liver damage. So, even if liver function test values double, you can't assume that the amount of diseased liver tissue has also doubled. To complicate matters, most hepatic tests measure functions the liver shares with other organs, such as enzyme production, or alterations associated with liver cell injury rather than liver function impairment. What's more, hepatic test results may be false positive or false negative.

To accurately assess your patient's condition, first take a thorough health history and perform a complete physical examination. Remember to ask about exposure to environmental chemicals. Also note any possible signs and symptoms of liver disease, such as poor resistance to disease, anorexia, chronic fatigue, muscle wasting, tendency to bruise eas-

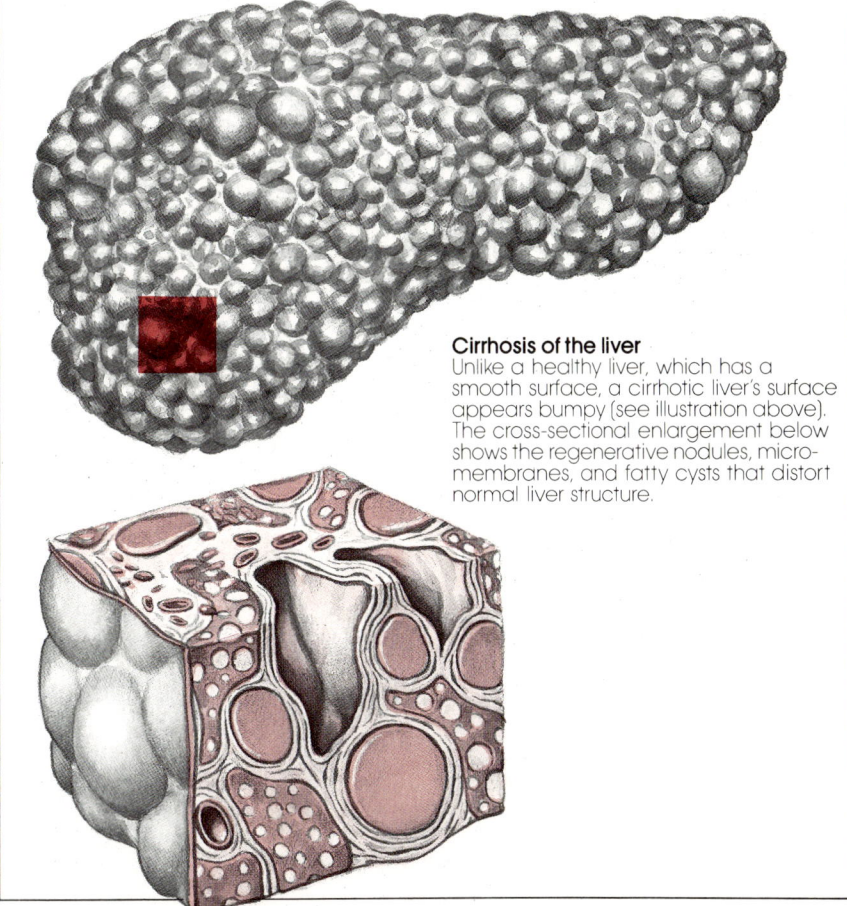

CONTINUED ON PAGE 80

Cirrhosis of the liver
Unlike a healthy liver, which has a smooth surface, a cirrhotic liver's surface appears bumpy (see illustration above). The cross-sectional enlargement below shows the regenerative nodules, micromembranes, and fatty cysts that distort normal liver structure.

MODIFYING DRUG THERAPY

LIVER DISEASE

DRUGS AND LIVER DISEASE CONTINUED

ily or bleed from mucous membranes, and a fetid body odor. Then, analyze hepatic test results in conjunction with your history and assessment findings. With this information at hand, you can make a fairly accurate assessment of your patient's liver function and determine whether ordered drug dosages are appropriate for your patient.

Ongoing assessment. Once your patient has begun drug therapy, liver function studies should be repeated frequently, so that you can monitor improvements or deterioration in liver function. Throughout your patient's hospitalization, use percussion and palpation to assess liver size. Monitor his mental status, watching especially for decreasing level of consciousness. And stay alert to physical signs of worsening liver disease, such as:

• *increasing jaundice.* In mild liver disease, some yellowing may appear in the patient's sclera, on the underside of his tongue, and at the back of his hard palate. As liver disease worsens, the skin and face of a light-complexioned patient becomes yellow.

• *spider angioma, red palms, dilated veins around the umbilicus, and engorged abdominal veins.* These signs may indicate cirrhosis of the liver with portal hypertension.

• *ascites and edema.* These conditions usually indicate advanced liver disease. As liver disease worsens, ascites becomes more severe.

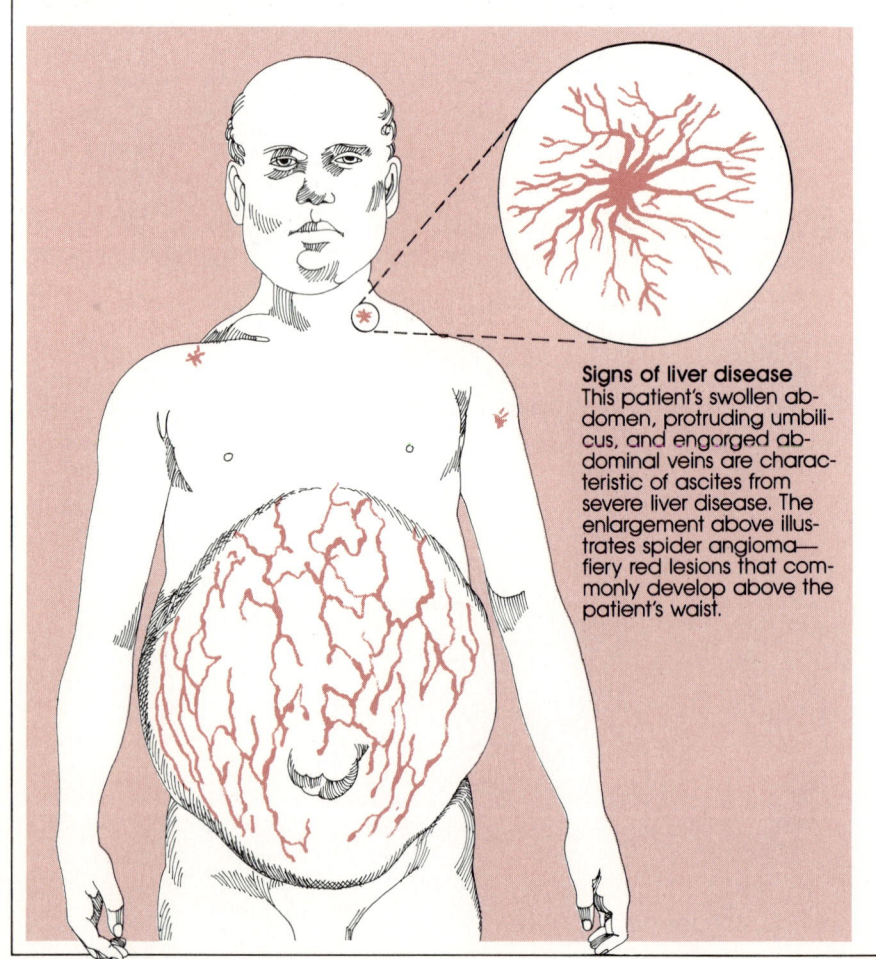

Signs of liver disease
This patient's swollen abdomen, protruding umbilicus, and engorged abdominal veins are characteristic of ascites from severe liver disease. The enlargement above illustrates spider angioma—fiery red lesions that commonly develop above the patient's waist.

THE LIVER PROFILE: ASSESSING LIVER FUNCTION

Any hepatic test a doctor orders reveals some information about your patient's liver function. To get the full picture, however, consider the results of several specific liver function tests. Together, these tests, which form the patient's liver profile, act as a fairly accurate gauge of his liver's ability to eliminate drugs.

You may hear liver profile tests called liver enzyme studies. As you'll see, the expression *liver enzymes* is really a misnomer because these enzymes are also found in other body tissues.

In most cases, a liver profile consists of the following tests:

Alkaline phosphatase. This enzyme is found in the liver as well as in bone, intestine, and kidney tissue. The liver normally excretes alkaline phosphatase in the bile. So increased serum alkaline phosphatase may be caused by the liver's inability to metabolize and excrete the enzyme. Or the elevated alkaline phosphatase may be caused by obstructive jaundice stemming from a blockage in the common bile duct.

Serum glutamic-pyruvic transaminase (SGPT). Although this enzyme is found in kidney, heart, and skeletal muscle tissue, it's most highly concentrated in liver tissue. So, even though SGPT values increase when these other tissues are damaged, elevated test values most strongly reflect liver damage. In a patient known to have liver disease, a markedly elevated SGPT level may indicate liver cell necrosis or destruction. *Note:* This test is also called alanine aminotransferase.

Serum glutamic-oxaloacetic transaminase (SGOT). This enzyme is found mainly in heart, kidney, liver, and muscle tissue and in red blood cells. In response to liver damage, SGOT

MODIFYING DRUG THERAPY

values rise prior to any sign of jaundice. Therefore, an elevated SGOT can indicate early liver dysfunction caused by liver cell injury or necrosis.

SGOT is less specific for liver damage than SGPT. Unlike SGPT, SGOT rises in the presence of heart muscle damage caused by myocardial infarction. *Note:* This test is also called aspartate aminotransferase.

Lactate dehydrogenase (LDH). This enzyme is found mainly in the heart, liver, kidney, brain, skeletal muscles, and red blood cells. It can be separated into five isoenzymes, two of which are specific to the liver (LDH_4 and LDH_5). Increased levels of these two isoenzymes suggest liver damage. LDH studies have less diagnostic value than other enzyme studies.

Bilirubin. A by-product of hemoglobin breakdown, bilirubin is metabolized and made water-soluble by the liver and is then excreted by the intestines as a component of bile salts. Elevated bilirubin levels can indicate either liver dysfunction or an obstruction of bile flow from the liver. The specific implication depends on whether the test identifies serum bilirubin as indirect (prehepatic) or direct (posthepatic):

Direct bilirubin. Water-soluble bilirubin reacts directly when reagents are added to the blood specimen. Therefore, when direct bilirubin levels are high, suspect obstructed bile flow caused by blockage in the liver's collecting channels, hepatic duct, or common bile duct.

Indirect bilirubin. This is free, nonmetabolized bilirubin, which only reacts to reagents when alcohol is added to the test solution. High levels of indirect bilirubin may indicate the liver's inability to conjugate the waste product.

Serum albumin. Albumin, a protein produced by the liver, serves several important purposes. First, albumin prevents body fluids from leaking into interstitial spaces and the peritoneal cavity. And it transports calcium through the bloodstream and drugs, lipids, and toxins (such as bilirubin) to the liver, where they're metabolized. A drop in serum albumin levels to 2.5 g/dl or less indicates that the liver will have difficulty metabolizing drugs. Serum albumin is a reliable indicator of the severity and prognosis of chronic liver disease.

Prothrombin time. Prothrombin, a plasma protein, is a clotting factor that prevents hemorrhage and promotes thrombus formation. The liver synthesizes prothrombin when sufficient vitamin K concentrations are present in the liver. Consequently, any impairment in the liver or in the liver's ability to utilize vitamin K will decrease prothrombin synthesis and interfere with the blood's ability to clot. Prothrombin time reflects the liver's ability to synthesize prothrombin.

Prothrombin time values can help you distinguish between bile duct obstruction and liver tissue damage. If clotting time is normal after vitamin K is added, rule out liver cell damage. In this case, decreased prothrombin synthesis is probably the result of an obstruction in the patient's bile duct that prevents vitamin K from reaching the liver. However, if the blood specimen clots slowly in the presence of vitamin K, decreased prothrombin synthesis is probably the result of liver cell damage.

PLANNING DRUG THERAPY: POINTS TO REMEMBER

If your patient has a liver disorder, expect his response to drug therapy to be unpredictable. Although continuing liver function studies may suggest an improvement (or deterioration) in his condition, they don't necessarily correspond to changes in liver function. Because test results are incomplete indicators, you must rely on your assessment skills to minimize the risk of adverse reactions.

Throughout your patient's hospitalization, administer all drugs with extreme caution and monitor his response carefully. In addition, keep these special considerations in mind:

• Liver failure alters the action of any drug that's primarily metabolized in the liver. Because unmetabolized drug molecules accumulate in the bloodstream, the patient may experience enhanced or toxic drug effects. The toxic effects of certain drugs—for example, analgesics, diuretics, and such CNS depressants as sedatives and anesthetics—can lead to hepatic coma in a patient with liver failure. Other drugs, such as digitoxin, can cause digitalis toxicity. Lidocaine and theophylline can also cause seizures in addition to other serious adverse reactions.

• Liver disease can alter a patient's sensitivity to certain drugs. For example, anticoagulants may increase his risk of bleeding as a result of reduced vitamin K absorption or decreased synthesis of clotting factors that require vitamin K. Some diuretics may cause excessive potassium loss in a patient with liver disease. This, in turn, may induce hypokalemic alkalosis. Because alkalosis permits ammonia to move into the bloodstream more easily, hepatic

CONTINUED ON PAGE 82

LIVER DISEASE

PLANNING DRUG THERAPY: POINTS TO REMEMBER CONTINUED

coma may result.
• Because liver dysfunction decreases glycogenesis, the patient's risk of hypoglycemia increases with the use of such drugs as tolbutamide, tolazamide, and acetohexamide.
• Liver disease can decrease albumin synthesis and cause albumin to leak into interstitial fluid. As a result, the patient is at increased risk of developing hypoalbuminemia. Because such drugs as prednisone, phenytoin, and diazepam have fewer protein-binding sites, they remain free (active) in the patient's system longer. This increases the patient's risk of drug toxicity.
• Altered drug effects are a major risk in the alcoholic patient with liver damage. *Chronic* alcohol ingestion induces hepatic enzymes, decreasing drug effects. But if the patient's plasma alcohol levels are high from *acute* alcohol ingestion, the alcohol competes with other drugs. In this case, other drugs may be metabolized more slowly, which enhances their effects.

Important: A number of drugs are known to be hepatotoxic. To prevent further damage to your patient's liver, avoid using these drugs. For examples of hepatotoxic drugs, see the list below.

HOW LIVER DISEASE AFFECTS DRUG ACTION

By slowing drug metabolism, liver disease enhances the effects of many drugs. This, in turn, increases the risk of adverse reactions and interactions.

For examples of high-risk drugs, examine the following list. Use caution when giving any of these drugs to a patient with liver disease.
• acetaminophen
• anticoagulants, oral
• barbiturates
• chloramphenicol
• chlordiazepoxide
• diazepam and prazepam
• digitoxin
• diuretics (especially potassium-losing ones)
• ergotamine
• hypoglycemics, oral
• lidocaine
• narcotics
• phenytoin
• prednisolone and prednisone
• propranolol
• rifampin
• theophylline

DRUGS AND LIVER TOXICITY

Drug-induced liver toxicity can be classified as either intrinsic or extrinsic. Here's how they compare.
Intrinsic hepatotoxicity is caused by hepatotoxic substances, such as chemical poisons or hepatotoxic drugs. Two types of injury can result: cytotoxic or cholestatic. *Cytotoxic* injury refers to necrosis of the liver's parenchymal cells. *Cholestatic* injury refers to obstructive jaundice from bile flow inhibition.

Some drugs known to cause intrinsic cytotoxic injury include alcohol, tetracycline (usually in I.V. form only), dantrolene, methotrexate, acetaminophen (in large doses), and rifampin. Drugs known to cause intrinsic cholestatic injury include chlorpropamide, oxymetholone, and niacin.
Idiosyncratic hepatotoxicity is apparently caused by drug hypersensitivity. Like intrinsic hepatotoxicity, idiosyncratic hepatotoxicity can cause either cytotoxic or cholestatic injury. Halothane, penicillins, phenytoin, valproic acid, and quinidine are several drugs associated with idiosyncratic cytotoxic injury. Erythromycin estolate and phenothiazines are associated with idiosyncratic cholestatic injury.

HEPATOTOXIC DRUGS: SOME EXAMPLES

The following drugs are known for their ability to cause liver damage. A patient with normal liver function who's receiving one of these drugs must be closely monitored with liver function studies. *Caution:* Don't give these drugs to a patient with preexisting liver disease unless no acceptable alternative exists and the potential benefits of drug therapy outweigh the risks.
• acetaminophen in high doses
• chlorpropamide
• dantrolene
• erythromycin estolate (Ilosone)
• halothane
• isoniazid (INH)
• ketoconazole
• methotrexate
• methoxyflurane
• mithramycin
• niacin
• nitrofurantoin (Macrodantin)
• oxymetholone (Anadrol-50*)
• penicillins
• phenothiazines
• phenytoin
• pyrazinamide
• quinidine
• rifampin
• salicylates in high doses
• sulfonamides
• tetracycline (I.V. only)
• valproic acid

*Not available in Canada

ACUTE CONDITIONS

How acute conditions affect drug action

How does an acute, life-threatening condition alter your patient's response to drug therapy? Although the full answer is complex, such a condition primarily affects drug action by altering liver and kidney function. As a result, the body's ability to metabolize and excrete drugs is impaired. Read what follows for guidelines.

CARDIOGENIC SHOCK (ACUTE HEART FAILURE)

Effects
Impaired hepatic blood flow, causing liver congestion and hypoperfusion. As a result, drugs are metabolized more slowly and may accumulate in the bloodstream, causing toxicity.

Nursing considerations
• Monitor the patient's response to drug therapy. As ordered, reduce drug dosages to prevent toxicity.
• When cardiac function improves and drug metabolism returns to normal, increase drug dosages, as ordered, to maintain therapeutic levels.

Note: The tissue hypoperfusion that accompanies shock reduces or delays absorption of drugs given intramuscularly. As ordered, give drugs I.V. whenever possible.

RESPIRATORY FAILURE

Effects
Hypoxemia, right ventricular heart failure (cor pulmonale), liver congestion, and renal failure from reduced blood flow to the kidneys

Nursing considerations
• As ordered, reduce drug dosages, especially of theophylline, a drug commonly ordered to treat bronchopulmonary disorders. Respiratory failure tends to prolong drug effects by impairing hepatic clearance and renal excretion.
• If the patient is on a ventilator, monitor him for altered response to drug therapy. Keep in mind that mechanical ventilation can reduce cardiac output. This, in turn, leads to hepatic congestion, decreased renal function, and fluid retention, which alters drug distribution, metabolism, and excretion.

BURNS

Effects
Reduced cardiac and hepatic function, impairing drug clearance. In addition, reduced serum albumin and third-space fluid shift impair protein binding and alter drug distribution. But loss of drug-carrying plasma can increase drug clearance. Likewise, loss of drugs in burn fluid (for example, aminoglycosides) can result in increased drug clearance.

Nursing considerations
• If the patient is receiving an I.V. antibiotic, monitor plasma drug values to determine peak and trough levels.

TRAUMA

Effects
Increased protein requirements for tissue repair, reducing plasma albumin levels and therefore protein-binding sites; reduced GI motility; tissue hypoperfusion

Nursing considerations
• Tissue hypoperfusion slows intramuscular drug absorption. As ordered, give drugs I.V.
• As ordered, reduce I.V. drug dosages. Because protein-binding sites are reduced, free drug levels rise.
• If ordered, increase dosages of oral or intramuscular drugs.

Note: Major surgery affects the body in much the same way as traumatic injuries. Narcotic analgesics administered perioperatively inhibit gastric and intestinal motility and cause urinary retention. During the early postoperative period, give drugs by the I.V. route, as ordered.

Predicting compliance

If your patient has a chronic disorder that requires long-term self-medication, his compliance is essential. By exploring his history and self-medication practices, you can probably predict how well he's likely to comply. Keep these factors in mind.

• *Family history.* Find out if any of your patient's relatives have been treated for chronic illness. You may discover, for example, that his mother died shortly after beginning digitalis therapy and that he now associates the drug with death.

• *Use of OTC products.* Generally, regular use of OTC drugs signifies confidence in drug therapy. But regular OTC use may also breed some misconceptions. A patient who regularly uses aspirin, for example, may be accustomed to fast pain relief. As a result, he could become disillusioned with a drug that requires days or weeks to take effect. Also keep in mind that a patient who's accustomed to self-medication may feel free to improvise with his drug regimen. Take extra time to emphasize the importance of following dosage instructions.

• *Preconceptions formed by the media.* Your patient may have his own ideas about how his condition should be treated. If necessary, emphasize that the popular media don't always reflect the latest medical findings.

• *Attitudes about drug therapy.* Finally, remember that your patient's receptiveness to your instructions hinges on his confidence that drug therapy will help him and on your credibility. Although some patients think that a pill can cure anything, others believe that relying on drugs is unnatural or a sign of weakness. If your patient feels this way, anticipate noncompliance.

MODIFYING DRUG THERAPY

LIFE-STYLE

DRUG THERAPY AND DAILY LIVING

"Mr. Markus, do you drink alcoholic beverages? About how many a day?"

Do you feel uncomfortable asking your patient such personal questions? If so, read the following pages for a reminder of how important his answers can be to the success—and safety—of drug therapy.

In addition to prescription drugs, your patient may be taking any number of over-the-counter products. But keep in mind that not all drugs are found in the pharmacy. Substances your patient eats, drinks, or inhales are also, in a broad sense, drugs— and they're capable of interacting with other drugs he takes.

Chances are, between work and home, your patient is exposed to some or all of these chemicals: carbon monoxide, cyclic hydrocarbons, halogenated hydrocarbons, heavy metals, ketones, nitrogen compounds, sulfur dioxide, and sulfuric acid. Even a simple task like spraying a rosebush for beetles exposes your patient to chemicals that could trigger a drug interaction.

When taking your patient's history, don't neglect to explore such matters as his eating habits, alcohol consumption, whether he smokes, and even the quality of the air he breathes at home or work. For details about why these life-style factors are so significant, read on.

TOBACCO SMOKE: INDUCER AND INHIBITOR

By now, everyone knows that tobacco smoke is linked to a variety of respiratory diseases, including lung cancer. But are you aware that smoking also affects the metabolism of certain drugs? Nicotine, one of the ingredients in tobacco smoke, is an enzyme inducer that may speed drug metabolism. Nicotine also increases corticosteroid secretion, which additionally induces drug metabolism.

Does this mean that a patient who smokes needs higher drug dosages than a nonsmoking patient? Not necessarily. Nicotine

The enzyme-inducing effect of nicotine tends to diminish with a person's age.

also frees fats from adipose tissue; these fats, in turn, may compete with drugs for protein-binding sites. Because smokers over age 30 tend to have lower serum albumin levels than nonsmokers, this factor may contribute to higher levels of free (active) drug. As a result, such a patient may need a *lower* dosage of a highly protein-bound drug.

Other noxious ingredients. In addition to nicotine, tobacco smoke contains such nongaseous matter as acids, alcohol, ketones, lipid-soluble polycyclic hydrocarbons, tars, and polyphenols. Among the gases contained in tobacco smoke are carbon monoxide, hydrogen cyanide, nitrous oxide, and nitrogen dioxide. All these substances affect drug action differently. Elevations in the blood's carbon monoxide level, for example, cause tissue hypoxia, which may *reduce* drug metabolism. Cyanide levels, however, appear to have little influence on drug metabolism.

In addition, tobacco smoke contains such toxic trace metals as cadmium, lead-210, and the radionuclide radium-226; and pesticides used during tobacco growing. These substances also affect drug metabolism in different ways. Cadmium, for instance, accumulates in the kidneys and liver, altering drug metabolism and excretion. Heavy trace metals, such as lead-210 and radium-226, may inhibit drug metabolism by inactivating enzymes. Halogenated hydrocarbon pesticides, such as DDT, tend to increase drug metabolism, while organophosphate pesticides inhibit metabolism.

Marijuana. Now that marijuana use is widespread, keep in mind that it too affects drug metabolism. Although extracted, purified cannabinoids tend to inhibit drug metabolism, *habitual* marijuana smoking enhances drug metabolism.

The bottom line. What do all these conflicting influences mean for your patient? As you might expect, no one has easy answers. The effects of smoking on drug action depend on such factors as the patient's age, diet, and physical condition, as well as the specific drug he's taking. Closely monitor your patient's response to drug therapy to assess the effect of his smoking on drug action. Document your findings and adjust drug dosages, as ordered.

Important: A nonsmoking patient who lives or works in a smoke-filled environment may face the same risk of smoke/drug interactions as a patient who smokes. Be sure to inquire about this life-style factor when you take his history.

PREGNANCY AND SMOKING

Is your patient who smokes also pregnant? Let her know she stands a greater risk of spontaneous abortion, stillbirth, premature delivery, early membrane rupture, and other complications that could be fatal to the infant she's carrying. And warn her that congenital malformations are also linked to maternal smoking.

Also emphasize that she's nearly twice as likely as a nonsmoking mother to give birth to an underweight infant. Infants born to smoking mothers tend to weigh 4 to 8 oz (0.1 to 0.2 kg) less than those born to to nonsmoking mothers.

Smoking and birth weight. How does smoking decrease birth weight? As the pregnant woman inhales and absorbs nicotine and carbon monoxide from tobacco smoke, her blood vessels constrict. Consequently, the flow of oxygen and nutrients delivered through her bloodstream to the fetus diminishes. The result: fetal growth retardation.

Smoking also interferes with the assimilation of certain nutrients essential to fetal growth. Deficiencies of calcium and vitamins C and B_{12} are common in smokers. Even mild maternal malnutrition in the last few weeks of gestation may impair fetal brain-cell division.

Why does low birth weight pose such a serious risk to an infant? For one thing, the underweight infant has a smaller liver, less subcutaneous fat and muscle, and reduced metabolic supplies. And he's especially prone to hypoglycemia because of his low glycogen stores. Severe hypoglycemia in a newborn can lead to permanent brain damage.

The underweight infant's problems don't end at birth. His future development could suffer, too. He may have learning and behavior disorders, mental retardation, cerebral palsy, epilepsy, or reduced adult stature.

Intervention. On her first visit, ask your pregnant patient if she smokes. If she does, try to persuade her to stop. Tell her how smoking can endanger her child's life or future well-being.

Obtain a thorough patient history. Keep in mind that your patient's pregnancy is at special risk if she's an older woman or if she has a history of perinatal loss, vaginal bleeding during a prior pregnancy, or anemia.

Ask your patient about her eating habits. If her nutrition is poor, explain how she can improve it.

To further encourage her to stop smoking, obtain expired carbon monoxide levels at each visit. Refer her to smoking clinics and support groups, as necessary.

If she hasn't stopped smoking by the end of the first trimester of pregnancy, tell her it's not too late to stop. Studies show that she can improve her chance of delivering a healthy infant if she stops smoking by the fourth month. If she can't stop, encourage her to reduce the number of cigarettes she smokes and to switch to a brand low in tar and nicotine.

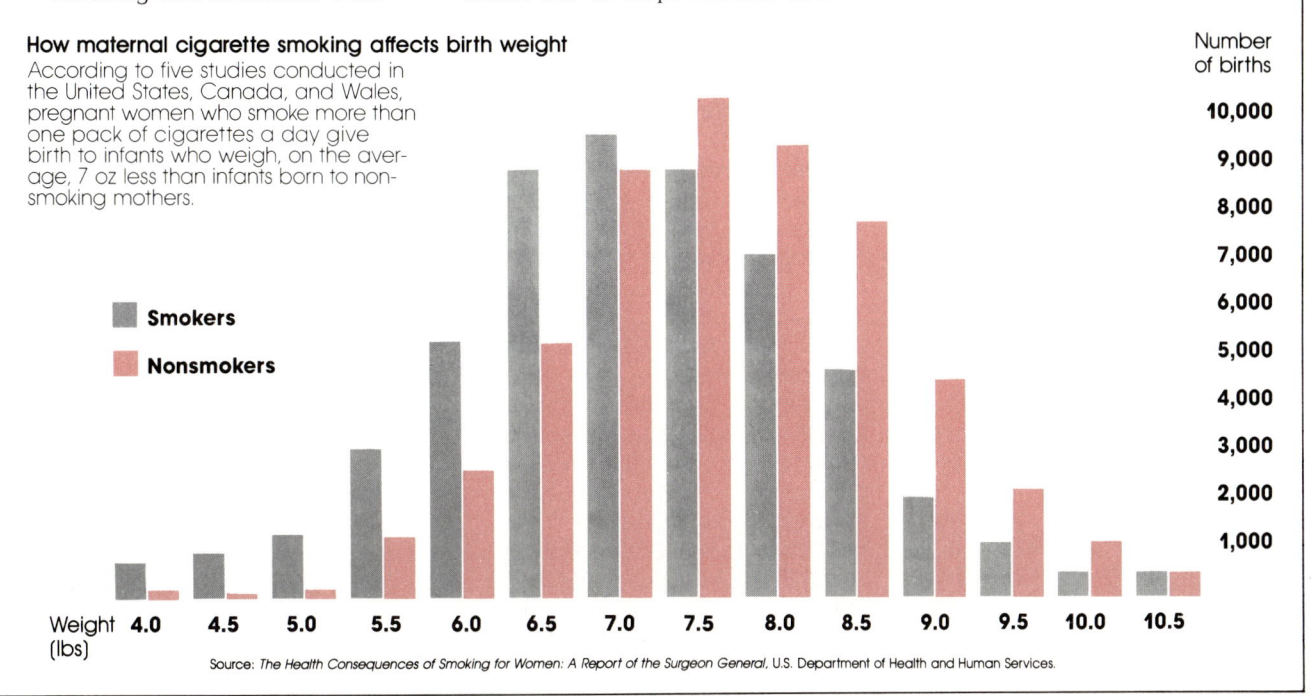

How maternal cigarette smoking affects birth weight

According to five studies conducted in the United States, Canada, and Wales, pregnant women who smoke more than one pack of cigarettes a day give birth to infants who weigh, on the average, 7 oz less than infants born to nonsmoking mothers.

Source: *The Health Consequences of Smoking for Women: A Report of the Surgeon General,* U.S. Department of Health and Human Services.

MODIFYING DRUG THERAPY

LIFE-STYLE

HOW SMOKING AFFECTS DRUG ACTION

Assessing your patient's condition or the effectiveness of his drug therapy? If he smokes, consider the possible effects of his habit on drug therapy. And remember, the same considerations may apply if he's constantly exposed to a smoke-filled environment.

The chart below identifies the effects smoking may have on a few drugs. When administering any of these drugs to a patient who smokes, continually assess his response. As ordered, closely monitor plasma drug levels and instruct him to report adverse reactions.

CNS DRUGS
Propoxyphene hydrochloride

Possible effects
- Increased drug metabolism, decreasing analgesic effects
- Reduced adverse reactions in some smokers

Nursing considerations
- Watch for a decrease in drug effectiveness.
- Increase dosages, if ordered.

PSYCHOTHERAPEUTIC DRUGS
Chlordiazepoxide hydrochloride
Chlorpromazine hydrochloride
Diazepam

Possible effect
- Decreased sedative effects

Nursing considerations
- Watch for a decrease in drug effectiveness.
- Adjust drug dosage, if ordered.

CARDIOVASCULAR DRUGS
Propranolol hydrochloride

Possible effects
- Increased drug metabolism, decreasing drug effectiveness. In addtion, smoking counteracts propranolol's effectiveness by increasing heart rate, stimulating catecholamine release from the adrenal medulla, raising arterial blood pressure, and increasing myocardial oxygen consumption.

Nursing considerations
- Monitor the patient's blood pressure and heart rate.
- Remember that propranolol-induced smoke/drug interactions may diminish as the patient ages.
  Note: To minimize this interaction, the doctor may substitute a selective beta blocker, such as atenolol.

HORMONES
Oral contraceptives containing estrogen and progestogen

Possible effects
- Increased adverse reactions, such as headache, dizziness, depression, libido changes, migraine, hypertension, edema, worsening of astigmatism or myopia, nausea, vomiting, and gallbladder disease
- Increased risk of myocardial infarction and thromboembolism

Nursing considerations
- Advise the patient of increased risk of heart attack and blood clots.
- Advise her to stop smoking or to use another birth control method.

VITAMINS
Ascorbic acid

Possible effects
- Low serum vitamin C levels
- Decreased oral absorption of vitamin C

Nursing consideration
- Encourage the patient to increase his vitamin C intake (especially if he's a heavy smoker).

MISCELLANEOUS
Theophylline

Possible effects
- Increased theophylline metabolism (from induction of liver microsomal enzymes) from smoking
- Lower plasma theophylline levels

Nursing considerations
- Monitor plasma theophylline levels and observe for lack of therapeutic effect.
- As ordered, increase theophylline dosage.

FOOD/DRUG INTERACTIONS: AVOIDING PITFALLS

"I usually take my medication with meals. Is that all right?"

If a patient asks you a question like this, you could conceivably respond with one of three answers: *yes, no,* or *maybe.* Of course, your response depends on many factors, including the specific drug prescribed and your patient's age and medical condition. But don't underestimate the importance of finding the *right* answer for him. In some instances, food/drug interactions mean the difference between the success or failure of drug therapy. To understand why, read the following information.

How food affects drugs. Food can influence drug absorption and action in several ways, according to the specific drugs and foods involved. In general, food delays dissolution and absorption of orally administered drugs. However, most drugs are eventually absorbed and the patient receives the intended therapeutic effect. But in some cases, food has an undesirable effect on therapy. For example, milk and dairy products can significantly reduce tetracycline's absorption. Calcium and magnesium ions in these foods chelate with the drug, reducing absorption by as much as 50%. As a result, the patient may fail to receive the intended therapeutic effect.

In other instances, food *enhances* drug absorption. By stimulating gastric acid secretion, for example, food in the stomach may enhance dissolution and absorption of acidic drugs.

Likewise, griseofulvin is best absorbed when taken with fatty foods. Because the drug is lipid-soluble, fatty foods accelerate the drug's dissolution.

But not all food/drug interactions involve drug absorption.

Some foods contain ingredients that can diminish a drug's therapeutic effect during distribution. For example, natural licorice made from the glycyrrhiza root contains an ingredient that, when eaten in excess over a long period of time, can elevate blood pressure and counteract antihypertensive drug therapy.

Food may contain natural or artificial chemicals that can interact with drugs. These interactions may limit a drug's therapeutic effect—or, in some instances, cause a life-threatening adverse reaction.

Similarly, *excessive* amounts of foods rich in vitamin K (such as liver and green, leafy vegetables) may antagonize an anticoagulant, diminishing the drug's effectiveness. That's why a patient taking an anticoagulant shouldn't drastically change his diet without his doctor's approval.

Although unusual, some food/drug interactions are life-threatening. The interaction between monoamine oxidase (MAO) inhibitors and foods containing tyramine is a classic example. When taken with such foods as aged cheeses, Chianti wine, or chicken livers, these drugs can trigger a hypertensive crisis.

How drugs affect nutrition. In addition to altering drug absorption and action, food/drug interactions can affect nutrition. Consider these examples:
• Cholestyramine can impair intestinal absorption of vitamins A, D, and K.
• Thiazide diuretics can cause severe potassium depletion. That's why a patient taking one of these drugs needs to eat plenty of potassium-rich foods, such as oranges, bananas, potatoes, and raisins.
• Oral contraceptives deplete the body of many vitamins, including folic acid and vitamin B_6.

Some drugs have a positive effect on nutrition. For example, ascorbic acid can enhance iron absorption.

Patient teaching. Encourage your patient to modify his diet to include foods rich in the vitamins or minerals depleted by the drug he's taking. Discourage him from trying to compensate for a poor diet with vitamin or mineral supplements.

Here are some additional points to teach your patient:
• Be sure to ask the doctor or pharmacist how the drug you're taking interacts with any foods or beverages you consume in large amounts. Report any unusual symptoms following the ingestion of specific foods to the doctor.
• Read the labels on over-the-counter drugs as well as package inserts included with prescription drugs. Follow these instructions closely.
• Follow the doctor's instructions concerning when to take drugs and what foods or beverages to avoid or include in your diet.
• Check with the doctor before making any major changes in your usual diet.

COPING WITH ENVIRONMENTAL HAZARDS

While your patient can avoid many potential drug interactions by modifying his life-style, he can't avoid all the environmental influences that could cause trouble. Every day, he's exposed to chemicals in the air he breathes, the water he drinks, and the land he inhabits. And some of these chemicals are physiologically active. In other words, they can alter drug effectiveness.

Agricultural chemicals, such as pesticides, are in the food your patient buys. And, as if agricultural chemicals aren't enough, industrial and residential chemicals (such as combustion gases from heating units and laundry detergent phosphates) put your patient at additional risk.

Some environmental hazards come from unexpected sources. A leaking microwave oven, for instance, can cause burns on a patient wearing a transdermal nitroglycerin patch.

How does all this affect you? Obviously, you can't eliminate environmental hazards—but you can help your patient cope with them. For example, advise a patient who jogs along a well-traveled highway to change his jogging route to a less-traveled path to reduce his carbon monoxide intake.

When you take your patient's history, take care to identify special environmental hazards. A patient who lives in the city usually inhales high amounts of carbon monoxide, while a farm dweller may ingest high amounts of pesticides.

Document your findings. That way, the doctor can consider environmental factors when prescribing a drug for your patient—and can increase or decrease the dosage, as necessary.

IDENTIFYING DRUG INTERACTIONS

Today, drug therapy has become remarkably complex. Potent and effective new drugs seem to appear on the market every week, while existing drugs are modified or combined to form new agents.

Because of these changes, your nursing responsibilities have grown. Not only must you know why and when each drug is used, but you must also learn how to safely administer drug combinations. Perhaps most important, you must be able to recognize signs that your patient's experiencing an undesired drug reaction or interaction and intervene appropriately.

How can you be sure you're giving your patient the best possible care when it comes to administering drugs? Let the charts in this section be your guide. On the pages that follow, you'll learn about specific drug interactions and possible adverse effects. You'll also find out which drug combinations to avoid and which to use with caution. In addition, you'll find easy-to-use guides to drugs that interfere with laboratory tests and cause incorrect test results.

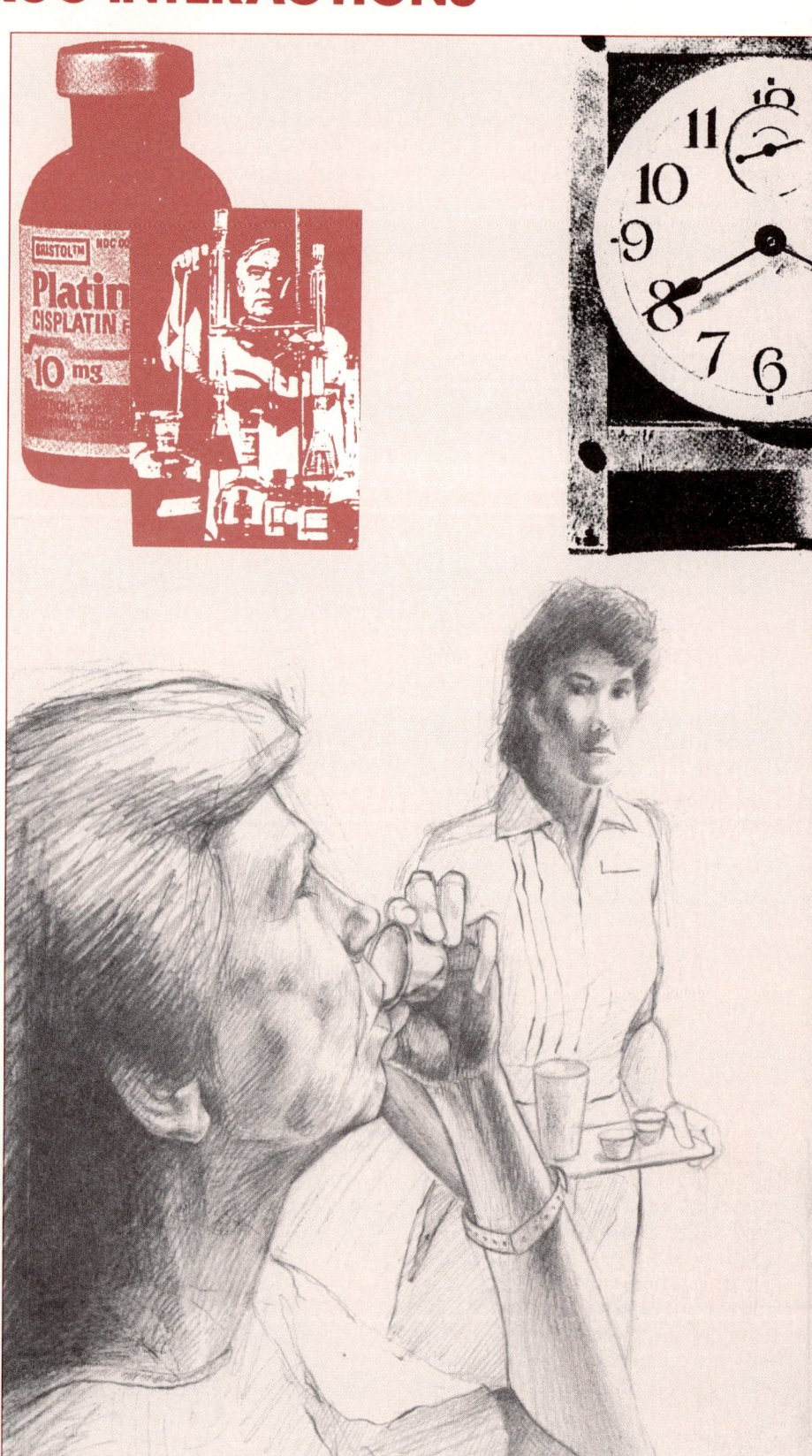

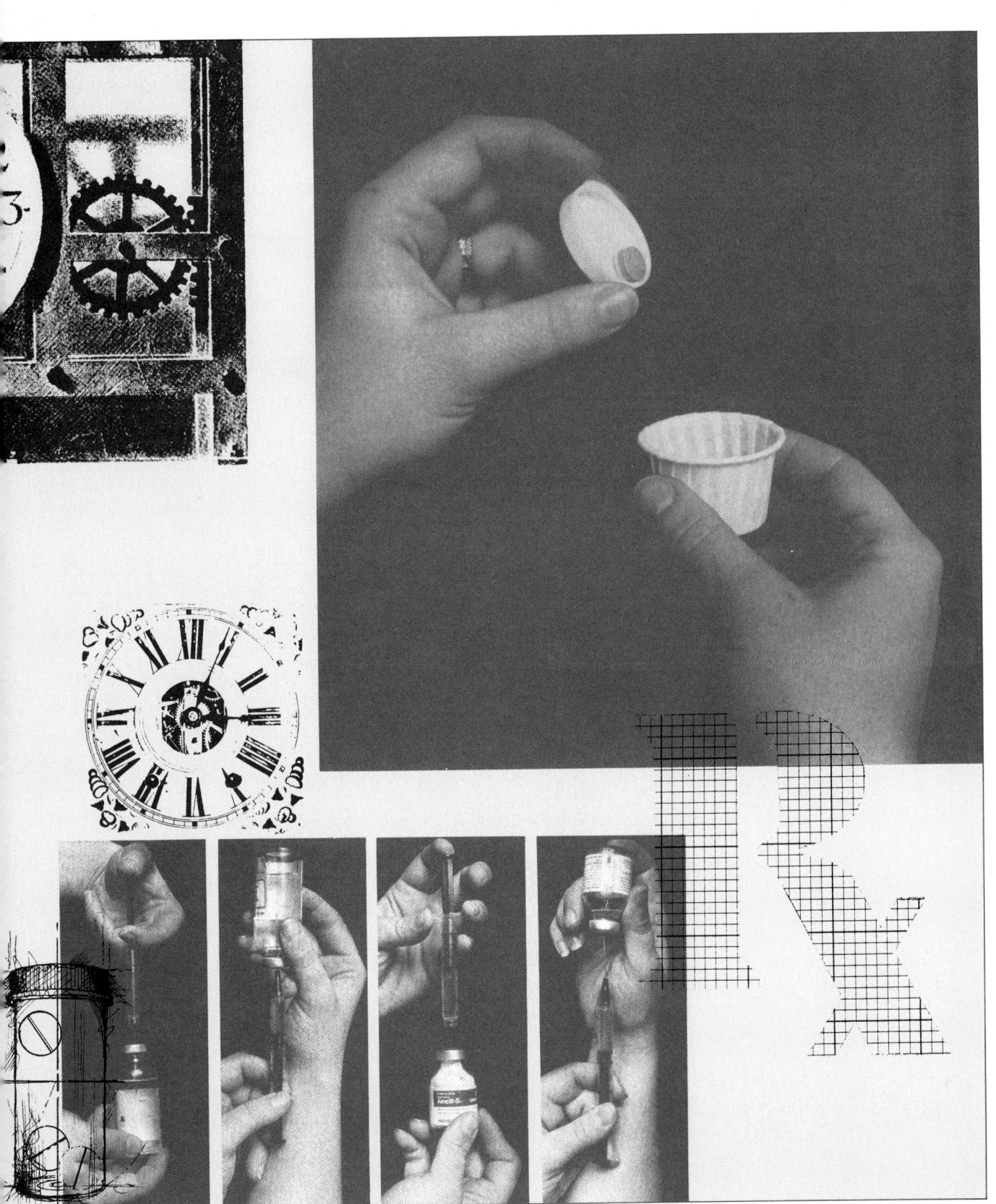

IDENTIFYING DRUG INTERACTIONS 89

YOUR ROLE

DEALING WITH DRUG INTERACTIONS

Do you feel confident when you administer medications to a patient who's receiving more than one drug? Or do you worry about the adverse reactions that a drug interaction may cause?

Even if you could keep track of all possible drug interactions, you'd have difficulty memorizing the possible dangers each combination poses. What's more, you know from experience that individuals vary a great deal in their responses to drugs. What's harmless to one patient may be perilous to another.

But don't assume that you must always avoid giving interacting drugs concurrently. Chances are, you can administer them together safely if you take appropriate precautions. The charts in this section will help you anticipate potential interactions between specific drugs and intervene correctly.

"Information about the existence or clinical significance of drug interactions changes rapidly—almost monthly. A drug once believed to be interaction-free may, after large-scale clinical use, warrant a drug-interaction warning. On the other hand, many drug interactions considered important in the 1960s and 1970s have proven to be much less significant than originally believed."

Larry N. Gever, RPh, PharmD
Springhouse, Pa.

Read the following information for general guidelines that apply when you give *any* drug combination.

Risk factors. Although you can't predict how a patient will respond to a given drug combination, you should be aware that certain risk factors predispose him to adverse reactions from a drug interaction. Ask yourself these questions:
• Does he have thyroid disease, diabetes, congestive heart failure, a GI disorder, or any chronic debilitating disease, such as liver or kidney failure? Is he an alcoholic? These conditions may affect drug absorption, distribution, metabolism, or excretion, so the patient has a greater chance of experiencing unwanted effects.
• Is he elderly? If so, his liver and kidney functions may be diminished, making him more vulnerable to the negative effects of a drug interaction.

Nursing considerations. Rarely is a drug interaction life-threatening. But a few combinations

HOW TO USE THESE CHARTS

On the following pages, you'll find drugs causing significant interactions organized in a logical, easy-to-read format. As you'll see, they're grouped by major drug category; for example, *Antiinfectives*. A few drugs that don't fall into a major category are listed on page 119 under *Miscellaneous Drugs*.

By using these charts, you can determine if the drugs your patient is taking have the potential to interact—and how to intervene if they do. To check a drug, use this book's index as your first resource.

If a drug you're checking isn't listed in the index, the reason may be that no well-substantiated

cause effects so severe that the doctor orders them only in unusual circumstances. And other combinations cause interactions that limit or prevent the intended effect of drug therapy. Check the charts in this section if you're in doubt.

If your patient experiences an unwanted reaction, notify the doctor. If the benefits of that particular combination outweigh the harmful consequences, he may adjust the dosage of one or both drugs, rather than discontinuing the combination.

In many cases, you can allay or even prevent the negative effects of an interaction by being thoroughly prepared for possible problems. Observe your patient closely and continue to do so throughout therapy—even if you don't notice anything unusual at first. Remember, some effects may not appear right away. Monitor laboratory test results, as ordered, and document any unusual signs or symptoms or unexpected reactions.

and clinically significant drug interactions occur. But double-check by also looking up the drug's major category. In drug classes containing many individual drugs, we've specifically named only those that are most frequently ordered. Interactions, however, often involve all members of the drug class.

Let's say, for example, that you're checking on cefaclor, a drug in the cephalosporin class. When you fail to find it in the index, check *cephalosporins*, listed on page 95 under *Antiinfectives*. There, you'll find that *all* cephalosporins interact with probenecid to elevate plasma cephalosporin levels.

IDENTIFYING DRUG INTERACTIONS

ANALGESICS

ANALGESICS: INTERACTIONS AFFECTING THERAPY

Can you anticipate a drug interaction involving an analgesic? The biggest obstacle could be your patient's failure to report the nonnarcotic over-the-counter pain products he uses. Because he can buy many of these products without a prescription, he may not consider them real medications and may overlook them when giving a drug history. Make a point of exploring this possibility.

When administering analgesics with other drugs, keep these other considerations in mind.

- Salicylates interact adversely with many drugs, including warfarin. Because salicylates are highly protein-bound, they can displace warfarin from its protein-binding sites. The result: more warfarin in the bloodstream and an intensified anticoagulant effect. (For more details, see page 98.) Similarly, if a patient takes aspirin while also taking probenecid for gout, he may get little gout relief. In continuous, low doses, aspirin has an antagonistic effect on the uric acid excretion that probenecid normally stimulates.
- Warn the patient who's taking a salicylate for its anti-inflammatory effect that large doses of antacids can hasten salicylate elimination, interfering with the salicylate's therapeutic effect.
- Be sure to keep a close watch on respiratory functions when caring for a patient receiving a narcotic analgesic and a barbiturate anesthetic. Additive respiratory depression may result from this combination.

SALICYLATES

All salicylates: aspirin, choline magnesium trisalicylate, choline salicylate, magnesium salicylate, salsalate, sodium salicylate, sodium thiosalicylate

Interacting drug	Possible effect	Nursing considerations
• Antacids (in large doses) - or - • Corticosteroids	Decreased salicylate effectiveness from hastened salicylate excretion	• Warn the patient against taking large doses of antacids. • To prevent possible GI distress, advise him to take aspirin with a glass of milk or with food. • Assess the patient to determine the effectiveness of aspirin therapy.
• Probenecid - or - • Sulfinpyrazone	Gout from increased serum uric acid levels; interaction blocks uric acid excretion	• Monitor serum uric acid levels. • Assess the patient for signs and symptoms of gout; for example, joint pain and inflammation, especially in the toes. Teach the patient to recognize and report gout symptoms. • Instruct the patient to avoid over-the-counter products containing aspirin. Also advise him to avoid alcohol and foods high in purine, such as coffee. These substances increase uric acid levels.
• Carbonic anhydrase inhibitors; for example, acetazolamide	Either salicylate toxicity or decreased salicylate effectiveness. Toxicity results from increased penetration of salicylic acid into the central nervous system. Decreased effectiveness results from alkaline urine, which hastens salicylate excretion.	• Watch for signs and symptoms of salicylate toxicity, such as hyperpnea, lethargy, vomiting, tinnitus, hearing loss, and dizziness. • Check for lack of salicylate effectiveness.

CONTINUED ON PAGE 92

ANALGESICS

ANALGESICS: INTERACTIONS AFFECTING THERAPY CONTINUED

NARCOTICS, OPIOID ANALGESICS, AND PROPOXYPHENE

All narcotics and opioid analgesics: alphaprodine, butorphanol, codeine, fentanyl, hydrocodone, hydromorphone, levorphanol, meperidine, methadone, morphine, nalbuphine, opium, oxycodone, oxymorphone, pentazocine

Interacting drug	Possible effect	Nursing considerations
• Barbiturate anesthetics (methohexital, thiamylal, thiopental)	Additive respiratory depression	• As ordered, give a lower dose of the narcotic analgesic (when administered with or a few hours before the barbiturate anesthetic). • Monitor the patient's respiratory rate.
• Cimetidine	Central nervous system toxicity and respiratory depression; mechanism unknown	• Monitor the patient's respiratory rate. • Be alert for signs of CNS toxicity, such as confusion and disorientation.

meperidine

Interacting drug	Possible effect	Nursing considerations
• Chlorpromazine	Additive respiratory depression	• Avoid this combination, if possible. • If these drugs must be given together, monitor the patient's respiratory rate.
• MAO inhibitors	Hypotension or hypertension, restlessness, and agitation; mechanism unknown. This interaction is uncommon but potentially fatal.	• Don't administer these drugs together.
• Phenytoin	Meperidine toxicity from increased meperidine metabolism resulting in formation of normeperidine, a potentially toxic metabolite	• Monitor the patient for signs of normeperidine toxicity, such as CNS excitation (tremors or twitches). • Decrease the meperidine dosage, as ordered.

IDENTIFYING DRUG INTERACTIONS

ANTI-INFECTIVES

ANTI-INFECTIVES: INTERACTIONS AFFECTING THERAPY

Most anti-infective drugs fall into one of the following classes: penicillins, cephalosporins, aminoglycosides, sulfonamides, tetracyclines, and antifungal agents. These drugs select their prey with care, penetrating and locking onto the pathogen while avoiding host cells.

Enhancing drug therapy. Doctors often prescribe anti-infectives in combination, to achieve an enhanced effect. For instance, you may administer penicillin and streptomycin to treat an enterococcal infection.

But when two anti-infectives have different mechanisms of action, the resulting interaction may defeat the purpose of therapy. Penicillin and tetracycline, for example, antagonize one another, diminishing the intended anti-infective effect of both drugs.

Special considerations.
• Drug interactions involving aminoglycosides can be among the most serious. These drugs can impair kidney function and hearing, even when used alone. If you must administer an aminoglycoside with another drug that's nephrotoxic or ototoxic, such as cephalothin or a loop diuretic, make sure you monitor the patient frequently for signs and symptoms of renal failure or hearing loss.
• Antacids can reduce the absorption of tetracycline and isoniazid. If the doctor orders one of these anti-infectives and an antacid, give the anti-infective either 1 hour before or 2 hours after the antacid.
• If your patient is just beginning anti-infective therapy while still receiving another drug, observe him closely for an acute initial reaction. For example, if you give erythromycin to a patient who's already receiving theophylline, watch for theophylline toxicity. This adverse reaction may develop rapidly because erythromycin blocks theophylline metabolism.
• If you have to adjust the dosage of one drug to offset the effects of its interaction with another, don't forget that the dosage will need to be revised when the anti-infective is discontinued.

ALL ORALLY ADMINISTERED ANTI-INFECTIVES

Interacting drug	Possible effect	Nursing considerations
• Warfarin	Bleeding; drug interaction reduces the population of intestinal bacteria that produce vitamin K, which is necessary for normal coagulation. As a result, warfarin's anticoagulant effect is heightened.	• Monitor prothrombin time for deviations from the desired value. • Monitor the patient's hemoglobin and hematocrit values. A decrease in these values may indicate bleeding. • Watch for bleeding or signs of occult bleeding; for example, ecchymotic areas, bleeding gums, nosebleeds, coffee-ground vomitus, hematuria, or melena. • Instruct the patient to keep appointments for regular laboratory tests. • Warn him against taking any over-the-counter drugs (particularly aspirin and antacids) without first checking with the doctor or pharmacist. Also instruct him to avoid alcohol. • Advise him against discontinuing any medication he was taking at the time warfarin therapy began, unless the doctor approves. • Encourage him to follow a normal, balanced diet. Tell him *not* to change his diet or increase his vitamin K intake without the doctor's approval. • Advise him to wear a Medic Alert tag indicating that he's taking an anticoagulant.

CONTINUED ON PAGE 94

ANTI-INFECTIVES

ANTI-INFECTIVES: INTERACTIONS AFFECTING THERAPY CONTINUED

AMINOGLYCOSIDES

All aminoglycosides: amikacin, gentamicin, kanamycin, neomycin, netilmicin, streptomycin, tobramycin

Interacting drug	Possible effect	Nursing considerations
• Cephalothin	Renal failure from additive nephrotoxic effects	• Monitor the patient's fluid intake and output. • Monitor renal function (blood urea nitrogen and serum creatinine values).
• Loop diuretics (ethacrynic acid, furosemide, and bumetanide)	Ototoxicity from increased antibiotic concentration in ear fluid (a synergistic effect); interaction also has the additive effect of increasing the ototoxicity of both drugs	• Monitor the patient for hearing loss. If possible, make sure that baseline audiometric testing is done and that testing is repeated once or twice weekly during therapy. • Regularly check the patient's hearing with a tuning fork, if available; or with a handier tool, such as a ticking watch. If using a watch, determine the distance at which he can no longer hear it tick. Then, note any differences in subsequent tests. • Teach the patient to recognize and report signs and symptoms of ototoxicity: hearing loss, ringing or a feeling of fullness in the ears, dizziness, clumsiness, severe headaches, and nausea or vomiting. Advise him to note how acutely he hears various sounds (music, conversation, and television, for example) and to report any changes to the doctor. • Regularly document hearing assessments.
• Neuromuscular blocking agents (nondepolarizing muscle relaxants, such as tubocurarine, atracurium, and pancuronium)	Neuromuscular blockade and respiratory arrest from additive or synergistic neuromuscular blocking activity	• Use these drugs together cautiously if the patient's renal or hepatic function is impaired. • Keep emergency resuscitation equipment on hand; neuromuscular blocking agents paralyze respiratory muscles. • Reduce the dosage frequency of the neuromuscular blocking agent, as ordered, according to the patient's response. • Monitor the patient for apnea. • Perform a baseline lung assessment by checking lung sounds and the rate, rhythm, and depth of respirations. Repeat the procedure frequently. • Monitor laboratory test results, especially arterial blood gas values, for changes in the patient's condition.
• Penicillins, especially carbenicillin (mixed in the same I.V. solution)	Failure to eliminate infection. When an aminoglycoside is mixed with high concentrations of a penicillin (especially carbenicillin) in an I.V. solution, the aminoglycoside becomes inactive.	• Don't mix aminoglycosides and penicillins together in the same I.V. container. Instead, give the drugs 1 hour apart. *Note:* In patients with impaired renal function, these drugs may interact despite this precaution. Monitor for decreased therapeutic effect. • Monitor peak and trough plasma aminoglycoside levels. • Assess the effectiveness of drug therapy in treating the infection.

CEPHALOSPORINS

All cephalosporins: for example, cefazolin, cefoperazone, cefoxitin

Interacting drug	Possible effect	Nursing considerations
• Probenecid	High plasma cephalosporin levels from decreased renal excretion of the anti-infective	• A cephalosporin may be given with probenecid to achieve higher plasma cephalosporin levels. • Use cautiously if the patient has impaired renal function.

cefoperazone, cefamandole, moxalactam

Interacting drug	Possible effect	Nursing considerations
• Alcohol	Antabuse-like reaction from inhibition of an enzyme called aldehyde dehydrogenase, causing acetaldehyde accumulation. *Note:* Other cephalosporins don't cause this interaction.	• Teach the patient to recognize signs and symptoms of Antabuse-like reaction: sweating, diarrhea, nausea and vomiting, and headache. • Instruct him to avoid alcohol, including over-the-counter drugs containing alcohol (for example, liquid cough and cold preparations).

PENICILLINS

All penicillins: for example, ampicillin, cloxacillin, penicillin G

Interacting drug	Possible effect	Nursing considerations
• Probenecid	High plasma penicillin levels from decreased renal excretion of the anti-infective	• A penicillin may be given with probenecid to achieve higher plasma penicillin levels. • Carefully document the patient's fluid intake and output. • Use cautiously if the patient has impaired renal function.

ampicillin

Interacting drug	Possible effect	Nursing consideration
• Allopurinol	Rash or other hypersensitivity reaction; mechanism unknown. *Note:* Other penicillins don't cause this interaction.	• Monitor the patient for rash or other hypersensitivity reaction.

CONTINUED ON PAGE 96

ANTI-INFECTIVES

ANTI-INFECTIVES: INTERACTIONS AFFECTING THERAPY CONTINUED

TETRACYCLINES
All tetracyclines: for example, doxycycline, oxytetracycline, tetracycline

Interacting drug	Possible effect	Nursing considerations
• Antacids containing aluminum, calcium, or magnesium - or - • Iron salts	Decreased absorption of tetracycline from chelation (combination) of tetracycline and metal	• Don't give tetracycline and an antacid simultaneously. Instead, give tetracycline 1 hour before the antacid or 2 hours after the antacid. • Instruct the patient not to take tetracycline with milk or milk-containing products and to avoid iron supplements.
• Penicillins	Failure to eliminate infection from mutual drug antagonism	• Give penicillin 1 hour before giving tetracycline.

OTHER ANTI-INFECTIVES
amphotericin B

Interacting drug	Possible effect	Nursing considerations
• Corticosteroids - or - • Diuretics	Hypokalemia from additive effects	• Obtain baseline serum potassium levels before therapy begins. Then, monitor serum levels at least twice weekly, especially if the patient's receiving a digitalis glycoside. Hypokalemia may cause digitalis toxicity. • Check serum potassium levels before giving diuretic doses. • Assess the patient for signs and symptoms of hypokalemia: muscle weakness or cramps, paresthesia, nausea or vomiting, rapid and irregular pulse, and ST segment depression on EKG. • Monitor his fluid intake and output. • Regularly assess bowel sounds; decreased peristalsis may accompany hypokalemia. • Instruct the patient to notify the doctor if he feels bloated or constipated or if he experiences any other possible symptoms of hypokalemia. • Encourage him to consume foods and beverages high in potassium, such as bananas and fruit juices.

erythromycin

Interacting drug	Possible effect	Nursing considerations
• Theophylline	Theophylline toxicity from decreased theophylline metabolism	• Regularly monitor plasma theophylline measurements and report rising levels. Therapeutic levels range from 10 to 20 µg/ml; higher levels may be toxic. • Assess the patient for signs and symptoms of theophylline toxicity: anorexia, nausea and vomiting, irregular heartbeat, confusion, muscle twitching, or seizures. Teach the patient to recognize and report these symptoms. • Warn the patient not to take any other drugs, including over-the-counter drugs, without the doctor's approval.

isoniazid

Interacting drug	Possible effect	Nursing considerations
• Antacids containing aluminum	Decreased antitubercular effectiveness from decreased isoniazid absorption	• Give isoniazid 1 hour before the antacid or 2 hours after the antacid.
• Carbamazepine	Increased toxicity of both drugs from a mutual synergism that produces a double-drug interaction	• Monitor the patient for increased liver enzymes, a sign of isoniazid toxicity. • Monitor for carbamazepine toxicity and increased plasma carbamazepine levels. Toxic levels are greater than 10 μg/ml (or as specified in your hospital's laboratory manual). Signs and symptoms of toxicity include dizziness, ataxia, stupor, and nausea and vomiting. *Note:* Carbamazepine toxicity may cause bone marrow depression.
• Corticosteroids	Decreased antitubercular effect from increased metabolism and excretion of isoniazid	• Monitor the patient for isoniazid effectiveness. • Increase the isoniazid dosage, as ordered.

metronidazole

Interacting drug	Possible effect	Nursing considerations
• Alcohol	Antabuse-like reaction from acetaldehyde accumulation	• Don't administer these drugs together. • Instruct the patient to avoid alcohol and over-the-counter drugs containing alcohol (for example, liquid cough and cold preparations). • Teach the patient to recognize and report symptoms of Antabuse-like reaction: sweating, diarrhea, nausea or vomiting, and headache.
• Disulfiram (Antabuse)	Acute toxic psychosis; mechanism unknown	• Avoid this drug combination, if possible. • If the patient must receive both drugs, closely observe him for signs of psychosis and notify the doctor immediately if they appear.

ORAL ANTICOAGULANTS

ORAL ANTICOAGULANTS: INTERACTIONS AFFECTING THERAPY

You've probably cared for a patient with a thromboembolism who required anticoagulant drug therapy. Remember how closely you monitored him, holding the next dose until you checked his latest prothrombin time results?

Ensuring effective but safe oral anticoagulant drug therapy is like walking a tightrope. The patient needs enough drug to prevent emboli formation, yet not so much that excessive bleeding results. And to complicate matters, the patient's probably receiving a variety of other drugs that may interact with the anticoagulant, resulting in potentially serious adverse reactions.

When administering oral anticoagulants, keep these points in mind:
• If your patient is taking warfarin concurrently with such drugs as phenylbutazone, quinidine, or cimetidine, monitor his prothrombin time as ordered and check for signs and symptoms of bleeding. These drugs tend to enhance warfarin's anticoagulant effect. *Important:* If necessary remind the doctor to order routine prothrombin values.
• Warn your patient to avoid taking salicylates (and over-the-counter preparations containing them) while on warfarin therapy, unless the doctor specifically approves this combination.
• If your patient is taking warfarin concurrently with carbamazepine, barbiturates, glutethimide, or rifampin, monitor him for signs of clotting. These drugs can reduce warfarin's effectiveness.
• When administering dicumarol and phenytoin, watch for bleeding *and* clotting. Phenytoin can either increase the risk of bleeding or the risk of clotting. (See page 100 for details.)
• Tell your patient to avoid foods high in vitamin K, such as cauliflower, spinach, and green tea. Vitamin K can counteract an anticoagulant's effects.
• Before the patient's discharged, schedule regular outpatient laboratory tests for him and instruct him to keep his appointments.
• Advise him to check with his doctor about sports participation.

WARFARIN AND DICUMAROL

Interacting drug	Possible effect	Nursing considerations
• Alcohol	Bleeding from additive hypoprothrombinemic effect, or decreased anticoagulant effect from enhanced warfarin metabolism	• Monitor prothrombin time for deviations from the patient's baseline value. • Monitor the patient's hemoglobin and hematocrit values. A decrease in these values may indicate bleeding. • Watch for bleeding and signs of occult bleeding; for example, melena, cloudy urine, or coffee-ground vomitus. • Instruct him to avoid alcoholic beverages in excess. Over-the-counter products containing alcohol, such as liquid cough and cold preparations, can be used with caution.
• Salicylates	Bleeding from displacement of warfarin from protein-binding sites and from additive hypoprothrombinemic effect	• Monitor prothrombin time. • Monitor the patient's hemoglobin and hematocrit values. A decrease in these values may indicate bleeding. • Watch for bleeding and signs of occult bleeding; for example, melena, cloudy urine, or coffee-ground vomitus. • Instruct the patient to avoid aspirin and over-the-counter products containing aspirin. • Tell him to report excessive or unexplained bleeding or bruising to his doctor.

IDENTIFYING DRUG INTERACTIONS

WARFARIN AND DICUMAROL continued

Interacting drug	Possible effect	Nursing considerations
• Carbamazepine - or - • Barbiturates - or - • Glutethimide - or - • Rifampin	Decreased anticoagulant effect from enhanced warfarin or dicumarol metabolism	• Monitor prothrombin time. • Watch for signs of increased clotting effect. • Adjust anticoagulant dosage, as ordered.
• Phenylbutazone - or - • Oxyphenbutazone - or - • Chloral hydrate	Bleeding from displacement of warfarin or dicumarol from protein-binding sites	• Use extreme caution when giving any of these drugs with an oral anticoagulant. • Monitor prothrombin time. • Monitor the patient's hemoglobin and hematocrit values. A decrease in these values may indicate bleeding. • Watch for bleeding and signs of occult bleeding; for example, melena, cloudy urine, or coffee-ground vomitus. • Notify the doctor if the patient develops GI distress or other signs that might indicate bleeding.
• Quinidine	Bleeding from additive hypoprothrombinemic effect	• Use these drugs together with caution. • Monitor prothrombin time. • Monitor the patient's hemoglobin and hematocrit values. A decrease in these values may indicate bleeding. • Watch for bleeding and signs of occult bleeding; for example, melena, cloudy urine, or coffee-ground vomitus.
• Clofibrate - or - • Disulfiram - or - • Thyroid hormones	Bleeding; mechanism unknown	• Monitor prothrombin time. • Monitor the patient's hemoglobin and hematocrit values. A decrease in these values may indicate bleeding. • Watch for bleeding and signs of occult bleeding; for example, melena, cloudy urine, or coffee-ground vomitus.
• Cholestyramine - or - • Colestipol	Decreased anticoagulant effect from decreased absorption	• Monitor prothrombin time. • Administer the drugs approximately 6 hours apart, if possible, to minimize the interaction.

CONTINUED ON PAGE 100

ORAL ANTICOAGULANTS

ORAL ANTICOAGULANTS: INTERACTIONS AFFECTING THERAPY CONTINUED

WARFARIN AND DICUMAROL continued

Interacting drug	Possible effect	Nursing considerations
• Acetaminophen	Bleeding if the patient takes more than 2.8 g of acetaminophen daily for more than 2 consecutive weeks; mechanism unknown	• If the patient is taking acetaminophen continuously at high dosage, monitor his prothrombin time and watch for bleeding and signs of occult bleeding; for example, melena, cloudy urine, or coffee-ground vomitus. • Monitor the patient's hemoglobin and hematocrit values. A decrease in these values may indicate bleeding. • Check the combination drug products your patient's taking, especially analgesics, for acetaminophen. *Note:* This interaction isn't significant if acetaminophen is taken only in the usual dosages recommended for relief of fever or pain.
• Androgens; for example, danazol, fluoxymesterone, and nandrolone	Bleeding from decreased production of clotting factors	• Monitor prothrombin time. • Monitor the patient's hemoglobin and hematocrit values. A decrease in these values may indicate bleeding. • Watch for bleeding and signs of occult bleeding; for example, melena, cloudy urine, or coffee-ground vomitus. • Reduce anticoagulant dosage, if ordered.

• Cimetidine
  - or -
• Metronidazole
  - or -
• Sulfonamides
	Bleeding from inhibition of warfarin metabolism in the liver	• Watch for bleeding and signs of occult bleeding; for example, melena, cloudy urine, or coffee-ground vomitus.
		• Monitor prothrombin time.
		• Monitor the patient's hemoglobin and hematocrit values. A decrease in these values may indicate bleeding.
		• Reduce anticoagulant dosage, if ordered.

DICUMAROL ONLY

Interacting drug	Possible effect	Nursing considerations
• Antidiabetics	Hypoglycemia or bleeding possibly due to displacement of either drug from protein-binding sites	• Monitor serum glucose levels and prothrombin time. • Monitor the patient's hemoglobin and hematocrit values. A decrease in these values may indicate bleeding. • Monitor food intake; supply snacks, if necessary.
• Phenytoin	Decreased anticoagulant effect from enhanced dicumarol metabolism, or increased anticoagulant effect. Also, plasma phenytoin levels may rise from decreased phenytoin metabolism.	• Monitor prothrombin time. • Monitor the patient's hemoglobin and hematocrit values. A decrease in these values may indicate bleeding. • Monitor plasma phenytoin levels. • Observe the patient for signs and symptoms of phenytoin toxicity: nystagmus, ataxia, slurred speech, and respiratory depression.

ANTICONVULSANTS

ANTICONVULSANTS: INTERACTIONS AFFECTING THERAPY

The most important point to remember when administering anticonvulsants is that these drugs have a very narrow therapeutic index. A small dosage increase can cause drug toxicity, while a small decrease can render it ineffective. And when you consider that many other drugs can interfere with the metabolism of an anticonvulsant, you can see why you'll need to monitor your patient very closely if he's receiving an anticonvulsant with another drug.

Phenothiazines, alcohol, and tricyclic antidepressants are among the drugs that can reduce the effectiveness of an anticonvulsant. If your patient must receive one of these drugs along with an anticonvulsant, take seizure precautions and check him frequently.

Carbamazepine is gaining wider use as an anticonvulsant. But because it's a potent liver enzyme inducer, it may speed the metabolism of another drug given concurrently and cause an undesirable interaction.

Phenobarbital, used as both an anticonvulsant and a psychotherapeutic drug, poses similar risks. To learn about additional interactions involving phenobarbital and other psychotherapeutic agents, consult the drug chart beginning on page 115.

Phenytoin has a high potential for drug interactions, too. Highly protein-bound, phenytoin is also a potent liver enzyme inducer. Make a point of becoming familiar with the therapeutic plasma levels of phenytoin as well as the signs and symptoms of phenytoin toxicity.

ALL ANTICONVULSANTS

Interacting drug	Possible effect	Nursing considerations
• Phenothiazines - or - • Tricyclic antidepressants	Increased risk of seizures from lowered seizure threshold	• Take seizure precautions. • Monitor the patient for development of seizures. • Adjust anticonvulsant dosage, if ordered.

CARBAMAZEPINE

Interacting drug	Possible effect	Nursing considerations
• Phenobarbital	Increased risk of seizures from increased carbamazepine metabolism	• Monitor plasma carbamazepine levels. Therapeutic levels range from 3 to 9 μg/ml.
• Erythromycin - or - • Propoxyphene	Carbamazepine toxicity from inhibition of carbamazepine metabolism	• Monitor plasma carbamazepine levels. • Adjust carbamazepine dosage, if ordered.

PHENOBARBITAL

Interacting drug	Possible effect	Nursing considerations
• Valproic acid	Phenobarbital toxicity; valproic acid inhibits phenobarbital metabolism	• Observe the patient for signs and symptoms of phenobarbital toxicity, such as sedation and drowsiness. • Monitor plasma phenobarbital levels. Therapeutic levels range from 15 to 40 μg/ml. • Avoid giving the patient other drugs that might depress respiratory function. • Advise the patient to notify the doctor before using alcohol or other drugs and before discontinuing the medications. Explain that because this combination may cause drowsiness, he should use caution when driving or operating machinery.

CONTINUED ON PAGE 102

IDENTIFYING DRUG INTERACTIONS

ANTICONVULSANTS

ANTICONVULSANTS: INTERACTIONS AFFECTING THERAPY CONTINUED

PHENYTOIN

Interacting drug	Possible effect	Nursing considerations
• Alcohol	Increased risk of seizures from a lowered seizure threshold and from stimulation of phenytoin metabolism	• Monitor plasma phenytoin levels. Therapeutic levels range from 10 to 20 µg/ml. • Monitor liver function test results for signs of hepatic damage. • Instruct the patient to avoid alcoholic beverages or over-the-counter drugs containing alcohol.
• Chloramphenicol, isoniazid, trimethoprim, and sulfonamides - or - • Cimetidine - or - • Disulfiram	Phenytoin toxicity from blocked metabolism of phenytoin	• Monitor plasma phenytoin levels. Therapeutic levels range from 10 to 20 µg/ml. • Check the patient for signs and symptoms of phenytoin toxicity, such as nystagmus and ataxia. • Monitor liver function test results for signs of hepatic damage. • Adjust phenytoin dosage, as ordered.
• Folic acid	Increased risk of seizures because folic acid increases phenytoin's metabolism and interferes with phenytoin's absorption	• Avoid this combination, if possible. If the drugs must be given together, increase the phenytoin dosage, as ordered. • Monitor plasma phenytoin levels. Therapeutic levels range from 10 to 20 µg/ml. • Take seizure precautions and observe the patient for signs and symptoms of phenytoin toxicity, such as nystagmus and ataxia.
• Oxyphenbutazone - or - • Phenylbutazone - or - • Valproic acid	Phenytoin toxicity from displacement of phenytoin from protein-binding sites	• Monitor plasma phenytoin levels. Therapeutic levels range from 10 to 20 µg/ml. • Check the patient for signs and symptoms of phenytoin toxicity, such as nystagmus and ataxia. • Monitor liver function test results for signs of hepatic damage.
• Levodopa	Decreased antiparkinson effect of levodopa; mechanism unknown	• Monitor the patient for signs and symptoms of decreased levodopa effectiveness, such as rigidity and tremors. • Increase levodopa dosage, if ordered. (Alternatively, the doctor may order another anticonvulsant that's not of the phenytoin type.)

ORAL ANTIDIABETICS

ORAL ANTIDIABETICS: INTERACTIONS AFFECTING THERAPY

Oral antidiabetics have made life easier for the adult-onset, non-insulin-dependent (type II) diabetic. These medications stimulate the release of natural insulin and increase the body's receptivity to insulin, thus eliminating the need for daily injections.

But an oral antidiabetic agent can spell trouble when administered with some other drugs. A sulfonamide, for example, may displace an antidiabetic drug from its protein-binding sites, causing hypoglycemia. Rifampin and chloramphenicol can alter the metabolism of an antidiabetic drug, producing toxicity or hyperglycemia.

Make sure to monitor serum glucose levels carefully if your patient is receiving a beta blocker concurrently with an oral antidiabetic agent. Beta blockers can inhibit the usual signs and symptoms of hypoglycemia and prevent rebound glycogenolysis. When this happens, serum glucose levels plummet and the patient may develop severe hypoglycemia—without experiencing any adrenergic warning signs, such as tachycardia, nervousness, and sweating.

When teaching your patient, stress these points.
• Warn him about the risks of drinking alcohol-containing beverages; he may be setting himself up for an Antabuse-like reaction. Oral antidiabetic drugs alter alcohol metabolism and cause acetaldehyde accumulation.
• Remind him that many over-the-counter cough and cold preparations contain alcohol. Tell him to check product labels and to avoid products containing alcohol.
• Advise him to wear a Medic Alert tag identifying his condition and the medication he takes.

ORAL ANTIDIABETICS

All orally administered antidiabetics: for example, acetohexamide, chlorpropamide, tolazamide, and tolbutamide

Interacting drug	Possible effect	Nursing considerations
• Alcohol	Antabuse-like reaction from acetaldehyde accumulation; also, possible hypoglycemia from additive effect	• Instruct the patient to avoid alcohol and over-the-counter products containing alcohol (for example, liquid cough and cold preparations). • Teach him to recognize the symptoms of an Antabuse-like reaction: sweating, diarrhea, nausea and vomiting, and headache.
• Beta blockers; for example, propranolol, nadolol, pindolol, and timolol	Hypoglycemia without the usual signs and symptoms. Beta blockers inhibit hypoglycemic signs and symptoms mediated by the adrenergic nervous system and may block rebound glycogenolysis	• Monitor serum glucose levels regularly. • Instruct the patient to adhere to his prescribed diet. • To minimize this interaction, the doctor may order a cardioselective beta blocker, such as atenolol or metoprolol.
• Chloramphenicol	Hypoglycemia from blocked metabolism of antidiabetic drugs	• Monitor serum glucose levels regularly. • Check the patient for signs and symptoms of hypoglycemia: sweating, confusion, pallor, and hunger.
• Oxyphenbutazone - or - • Phenylbutazone	Hypoglycemia from displacement of antidiabetic from protein-binding sites and possibly from inhibited excretion	• Avoid these combinations, if possible. • Closely monitor serum glucose levels. • Observe the patient for signs and symptoms of hypoglycemia.

CONTINUED ON PAGE 104

ORAL ANTIDIABETICS

ORAL ANTIDIABETICS: INTERACTIONS AFFECTING THERAPY CONTINUED

ORAL ANTIDIABETICS continued
All orally administered antidiabetics: for example, acetohexamide, chlorpropamide, tolazamide, and tolbutamide

Interacting drug	Possible effect	Nursing considerations
• Rifampin	Hyperglycemia and poor control of diabetes from increased metabolism of antidiabetic drug	• Monitor serum glucose levels. • Test urine for glucose and acetone regularly. • Check the patient for signs and symptoms of hyperglycemia: anorexia, nausea and vomiting, lethargy, thirst, and polyuria. • Tell him to avoid over-the-counter products containing sugar.
• Sulfonamides	Hypoglycemia, mainly from displacement of antidiabetic drug from protein-binding sites	• Monitor serum glucose levels. • Observe the patient for signs and symptoms of hypoglycemia: sweating, confusion, pallor, and hunger.
• Fenfluramine	Hypoglycemia from additive effect	• Monitor serum glucose levels. • Observe the patient for signs and symptoms of hypoglycemia: sweating, confusion, pallor, and hunger.
• MAO inhibitors - or - • Salicylates (in high doses)	Hypoglycemia; mechanism unknown	• Monitor serum glucose levels. • Observe the patient for signs and symptoms of hypoglycemia: sweating, confusion, pallor, and hunger.
• Dicumarol	Hypoglycemia or bleeding from displacement of either drug from protein-binding sites	• Monitor serum glucose levels and prothrombin time.
• Thiazide diuretics	Thiazide-produced hyperglycemia, which antagonizes antidiabetic action	• Monitor serum glucose levels. • Test urine for glucose and acetone regularly. • Observe the patient for signs and symptoms of hyperglycemia: anorexia, nausea and vomiting, lethargy, thirst, and polyuria.

10-DAY FREE TRIAL

Use the card on the right to:

1. Save **$2.00** on **each** book you purchase by subscribing to the NURSING NOW™ series.

—OR—

2. Buy *Drug Interactions* without subscribing to the series (and pay just $13.95).

Mail the postage-paid card at right ▶

The only journal that helps you cope with your *whole life* as a nurse.

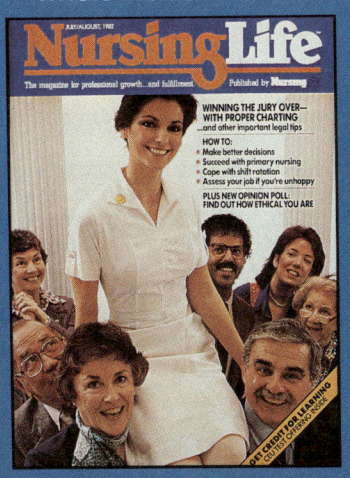

Give this card to a colleague.

Please check appropriate box.

☐ **YES.** I want to subscribe to the NURSING NOW series. Please send me *Drug Interactions* as my first volume. If I decide to keep it, I will pay just $11.95, plus shipping and handling. I understand that I will receive an exciting new NURSING NOW book approximately every other month on the same 10-day, free-examination basis. There is no minimum number of books I must buy, and I may cancel my subscription at any time by notifying you.

NB5S

☐ I want to buy *Drug Interactions* without joining the series. I will pay $13.95, plus shipping and handling for each copy. Please send me _____ copies and bill me.

5NB

Name _____
Address _____
City _____
State _____ Zip _____
Offer valid in U.S. only.   Prices subject to change.

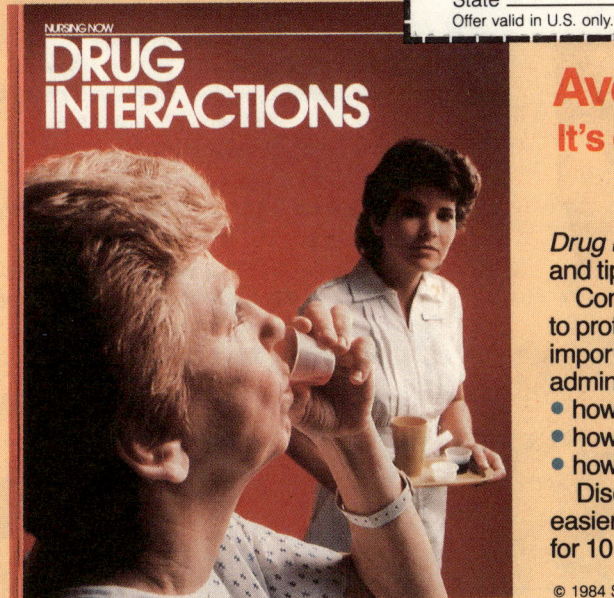

Avoid harmful drug interactions.
It's easier than ever, with this new book from the editors of *Nursing84 Books.*™

Drug Interactions is packed with advice on proper administration and tips to help you prevent dangerous drug interactions.

Comprehensive and easy-to-understand, this book tells you how to protect your patient from harmful drug effects and—just as important—how to protect yourself against the legal risks of administering drugs. You'll learn:
- how and why drug interactions occur
- how to avoid interactions
- how to make interactions less harmful when they're unavoidable.

Discover how this new book makes avoiding drug interactions easier than ever. Send for *Drug Interactions* today. Examine it FREE for 10 full days.

© 1984 Springhouse Corporation

Join those who are making *NursingLife* the fastest-growing nursing journal in the world.

FOR YOU OR A COLLEAGUE.

Your subscription to *NursingLife* will bring you down-to-earth solutions to the difficult people problems you encounter every day—on or off duty. You'll discover how to solve problems nursing school never covered: working with an incompetent doctor, the supervisor drinking on the job, colleagues abusing drugs, relatives asking advice. You'll see how to avoid malpractice suits, and so much more. Act today. Bring *NursingLife* into *your* life by taking advantage of this special get-acquainted offer: Receive 2 years (12 issues) of *NursingLife* PLUS a bonus issue for just **$15.95**...a savings of $20.05 over single-issue costs! You can cancel your subscription at any time and receive a refund for the unused portion of your payment. Your satisfaction is guaranteed.

☐ **Yes!** Send me 2 years of *NursingLife* for $15.95—plus my bonus issue.

Name _____
Address _____
City _____
State _____ Zip _____
I am an ☐ RN ☐ LPN ☐ Other. Do you now work in a hospital? ☐ Yes ☐ No

RNNA-6
Offer valid in U.S. only.

NursingLife is published bimonthly. Single copy price is $3 each, $18 a year.

BUSINESS REPLY CARD
FIRST CLASS PERMIT NO 2331 HICKSVILLE, N.Y.

POSTAGE WILL BE PAID BY ADDRESSEE

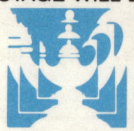

Springhouse Book Company
6 Commercial Street
Hicksville, N.Y. 11801

NO POSTAGE NECESSARY IF MAILED IN THE UNITED STATES

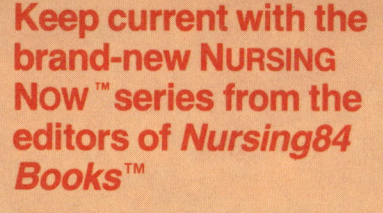

Keep current with the brand-new NURSING NOW™ series from the editors of *Nursing84 Books*™

The new NURSING NOW books help you cope with the nursing information explosion:
- new, complex procedures
- new, sophisticated drugs
- new technological advances
- new diagnostic tests
- new nursing considerations you must know to protect yourself legally.

Overwhelming? Not when you have NURSING NOW books to rely on. You'll find something new and useful on every page. And each page is designed to let you zero in on what you need to know...when you need to know it. Each volume is written in short, easy-to-digest modular units. Illustrations, charts, tables, and graphs let you get the most amount of information in the least amount of time. As a subscriber, you're entitled to examine each book in the NURSING NOW series for 10 full days **absolutely free!**

There's something new and useful on every page of every volume!

The series that keeps you up to date on the latest advances in nursing.

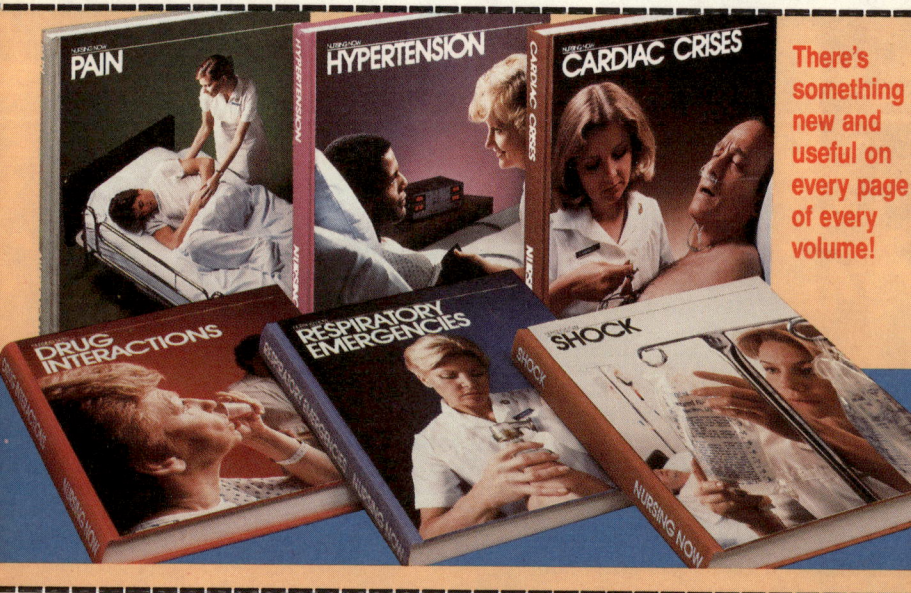

BUSINESS REPLY MAIL
FIRST CLASS PERMIT NO. 635, MARION, OHIO 43306

POSTAGE WILL BE PAID BY ADDRESSEE

NursingLife®
10 Health Care Circle
P.O. Box 1961
Marion, Ohio 43306

NO POSTAGE NECESSARY IF MAILED IN THE UNITED STATES

Mail this postage-paid card today to put the very next issue of NursingLife® to work for you.

A wealth of experience you can bank on:
- What to do when the doctor's wrong
- How to handle overwhelming stress
- How to cope with the pressure of constantly mushrooming new technology
- How to avoid legal trouble

Learn from the experience of nurses from around the world.

NursingLife listens to *you*...
talks to *you*...
cares about *you*...

From the publisher of *Nursing84®*

ANTINEOPLASTICS

ANTINEOPLASTICS: INTERACTIONS AFFECTING THERAPY

If you've ever cared for a patient receiving an antineoplastic drug, you're familiar with the adverse reactions these powerful drugs can produce. In addition to causing toxicity, they can:
• depress white blood cell production, increasing the risk of infection
• depress platelet production, increasing the risk of bleeding
• raise uric acid levels, exacerbating preexisting gout.

If you're giving other drugs to a patient on antineoplastic therapy, your main concern is to avoid drug interactions that could compound these adverse effects. And even over-the-counter products can be hazardous. If your patient's taking methotrexate, for example, aspirin can increase his risk of toxicity by displacing methotrexate from protein-binding sites and blocking its excretion.

As a rule, antineoplastic drug therapy is given periodically. Check your patient's drug schedule closely before he begins a new antineoplastic drug regimen, so you can anticipate potentially serious interactions.

AZATHIOPRINE AND MERCAPTOPURINE

Interacting drug	Possible effect	Nursing considerations
• Allopurinol	Increased hematologic toxicity leading to bleeding or infection from inhibited metabolism of azathioprine or mercaptopurine	• Decrease azathioprine or mercaptopurine dosage by one quarter to one third, as ordered. • Monitor hemoglobin and hematocrit values, and white blood cell (WBC) and platelet counts.

METHOTREXATE

Interacting drug	Possible effect	Nursing considerations
• Salicylates	Increased hematologic toxicity leading to bleeding or infection; salicylates prevent renal excretion of methotrexate and displace methotrexate from protein-binding sites	• Monitor hemoglobin and hematocrit values and WBC and platelet counts every 2 to 3 weeks. • Tell the patient to avoid over-the-counter products containing aspirin or other salicylates.
• Probenecid	Increased hematologic toxicity leading to bleeding or infection from inhibited renal excretion of methotrexate	• Decrease methotrexate dosage, as ordered. • Monitor hemoglobin and hematocrit values and WBC and platelet counts every 2 to 3 weeks. A decrease in hemoglobin and hematocrit values or platelet count may indicate bleeding. An increase in WBC count may indicate an infection.

PROCARBAZINE

Interacting drug	Possible effect	Nursing considerations
• Alcohol	Antabuse-like reaction from acetaldehyde accumulation, and additive CNS depression	• Tell the patient to avoid alcohol and over-the-counter products containing alcohol. • If he's consumed alcohol, observe him for excessive sedation.

IDENTIFYING DRUG INTERACTIONS

CARDIOVASCULAR DRUGS

CARDIOVASCULAR DRUGS: INTERACTIONS AFFECTING THERAPY

In many cases, drugs within this large category are administered together for therapeutic reasons. For instance, a patient with cardiac dysrhythmias may receive both a beta blocker and a calcium channel blocker in addition to an antiarrhythmic drug. Likewise, the doctor may prescribe diuretics along with a digitalis glycoside for treatment of congestive heart failure. Or, to relieve angina, he may order both a beta blocker and a calcium channel blocker.

But these combinations may lead to an interaction that produces undesirable effects. Here are some special considerations for a few cardiovascular drug types.

Antihypertensives. Of all cardiovascular drugs, antihypertensives are probably the most widely used. These drugs are commonly prescribed in combinations of two or more to take advantage of each drug's different mechanism of action. The intended therapeutic result is an increased antihypertensive effect with minimal adverse reactions. Unfortunately, antihypertensives may interact adversely with many other drugs, complicating drug therapy.

A wide range of drugs—including levodopa, tricyclic antidepressants, and phenothiazines—can curb the effectiveness of an antihypertensive drug. Knowing this, you can take steps to determine whether your patient's drug therapy is safe and effective.

A combination worth avoiding entirely is the antihypertensive drug guanethidine with a sympathomimetic agent, such as dopamine or norepinephrine. These drugs can interact to cause severe hypertension. And warn the patient who's receiving guanethidine to avoid over-the-counter products containing sympathomimetics, too.

Beta blockers. If your patient's receiving a beta blocker while taking an antidiabetic medication, monitor his serum glucose levels. Beta blockers can mask the normal signs and symptoms of hypoglycemia.

Calcium channel blockers. Verapamil, nifedipine, and diltiazem have become increasingly important in the treatment of angina and dysrhythmias. But healthcare professionals have discovered that these drugs can produce potentially hazardous interactions. Of the three drugs, verapamil is most likely to cause dangerous interactions. Consult this chart for details on these and other cardiovascular drugs.

ANTIARRHYTHMICS
lidocaine

Interacting drug	Possible effect	Nursing considerations
• Disopyramide - or - • Phenytoin	Myocardial depression, congestive heart failure, and dysrhythmias from additive effect	• Observe the patient for signs and symptoms of myocardial depression (such as hypotension and bradycardia), congestive heart failure, and dysrhythmias. • Obtain regular EKG readings, as ordered.
• Beta adrenergic blockers - or - • Cimetidine	Lidocaine toxicity from inhibited lidocaine metabolism	• Observe the patient for signs and symptoms of lidocaine toxicity, such as sedation, confusion, and seizures. • Also check for signs and symptoms of myocardial depression (such as hypotension and bradycardia), congestive heart failure, and dysrhythmias. • Monitor plasma lidocaine levels.
• Neuromuscular blocking agents; for example, succinylcholine	Increased neuromuscular blocking effect, causing prolonged respiratory depression; mechanism unknown	• Provide mechanical respiratory support, as required. • Closely monitor the patient for respiratory depression and apnea.

IDENTIFYING DRUG INTERACTIONS

quinidine

Interacting drug	Possible effect	Nursing considerations
• Drugs that alter urine pH; for example, vitamin C and carbonic anhydrase inhibitors, such as acetazolamide and antacids	Quinidine toxicity, causing myocardial depression and dysrhythmias, from urine alkalinization that increases quinidine reabsorption; or decreased quinidine effectiveness from urine acidification that decreases reabsorption	• Monitor urine pH and plasma quinidine levels. Therapeutic plasma levels range from 1 to 6 μg/ml. • Regularly check the patient's pulse and blood pressure. • Monitor his EKG readings for widening QRS complex and dysrhythmias • Teach the patient how to test his urine pH at home.
• Cimetidine	Quinidine toxicity from inhibited quinidine metabolism	• Monitor plasma quinidine levels. Therapeutic levels range from 1 to 6 μg/ml. • Regularly check the patient's pulse and blood pressure. • Monitor his EKG readings for widening QRS complex and dysrhythmias. • Adjust quinidine dosage, if ordered.
• Barbiturates - or - • Phenytoin - or - • Rifampin	Decreased quinidine effect from increased quinidine metabolism	• Monitor plasma quinidine levels. Therapeutic levels range from 1 to 6 μg/ml. • Regularly check the patient's pulse and blood pressure. • Monitor his EKG readings for widening QRS complex and dysrhythmias. • Assess the effectiveness of quinidine therapy.
• Neuromuscular blocking agents; for example, succinylcholine	Increased neuromuscular blocking effect, causing prolonged respiratory depression; mechanism unknown	• Provide mechanical respiratory support, as required. • Closely monitor the patient for respiratory depression and apnea. • Regularly check the patient's pulse and blood pressure. • Monitor his EKG readings for widening QRS complex and dysrhythmias.

ANTIHYPERTENSIVES

All antihypertensives causing orthostatic hypotension: for example, sympatholytic drugs

Interacting drug	Possible effect	Nursing considerations
• Phenothiazines; for example, chlorpromazine and prochlorperazine - or - • Nitrates; for example, nitroglycerin and isosorbide dinitrate	Orthostatic hypotension from additive hypotensive effect	• Monitor the patient for orthostatic changes in blood pressure and pulse while he's lying, sitting, and standing. • Advise the patient to stand slowly to avoid dizziness. • Administer nitrates while the patient is lying down to avoid severe headache and symptomatic hypotension.

CONTINUED ON PAGE 108

CARDIOVASCULAR DRUGS

CARDIOVASCULAR DRUGS: INTERACTIONS AFFECTING THERAPY CONTINUED

ANTIHYPERTENSIVES continued

captopril

Interacting drug	Possible effect	Nursing considerations
• Potassium or potassium-sparing diuretics (spironolactone, trimaterene, and amiloride)	Hyperkalemia from potassium retention caused by captopril	• Regularly monitor serum potassium and other electrolyte levels. • Monitor EKG readings for widening of QRS complexes, tall T waves, and ventricular fibrillation. • Check for other signs and symptoms of hyperkalemia: irritability, nausea, and diarrhea.
• Nonsteroidal anti-inflammatory agents; for example, indomethacin and ibuprofen	Reduced antihypertensive effect from inhibition of endogenous prostaglandin synthesis	• Monitor the patient's blood pressure carefully for worsening hypertension. If this occurs, the doctor may discontinue the anti-inflammatory agent.

clonidine

Interacting drug	Possible effect	Nursing considerations
• Levodopa	Reduced antiparkinsonian effectiveness from negation of levodopa activity	• Check for signs and symptoms of parkinsonism: facial grimacing, jerky arm and leg movements, and bobbing head. • As ordered, gradually discontinue clonidine over 24 hours and replace with another antihypertensive drug.
• Tricyclic antidepressants	Decreased antihypertensive effectiveness; mechanism unknown	• Monitor the patient's blood pressure carefully. • Emphasize the importance of having his blood pressure checked regularly after he leaves the hospital. • Adjust the clonidine dosage, as ordered.

guanethidine

Interacting drug	Possible effect	Nursing considerations
• Tricyclic antidepressants - or - • Amphetamines and amphetamine-like drugs; for example, fenfluramine - or - • Phenothiazines - or - • Haloperidol	Decreased antihypertensive effectiveness from inhibition of guanethidine's neuronal uptake	• Avoid these drug combinations, if possible. • If the doctor orders such a combination, suggest that he increase the guanethidine dosage. • Monitor the patient's blood pressure carefully. • Emphasize the importance of having his blood pressure checked regularly after he leaves the hospital.
• Sympathomimetics; for example, dopamine, ephedrine, phenylephrine, and norepinephrine	Severe hypertension from drug antagonism that reduces guanethidine's effectiveness, and increased sympathetic stimulation	• Avoid this drug combination. • Warn the patient taking guanethidine to avoid over-the-counter products containing sympathomimetics. Advise him to consult the pharmacist before using any over-the-counter product.

prazosin		
Interacting drug	**Possible effect**	**Nursing considerations**
• Beta adrenergic blockers	Acute hypotension from synergistic increase in prazosin effects	• Monitor the patient carefully for acute hypotension, especially following the first prazosin dose. First dose should be given at bedtime. • Emphasize the importance of having his blood pressure checked regularly after he leaves the hospital.

BETA ADRENERGIC BLOCKERS

All beta adrenergic blockers: atenolol, metoprolol, nadolol, pindolol, propranolol, timolol

Interacting drug	Possible effect	Nursing considerations
• All bronchodilators; for example, albuterol, aminophylline, metaproterenol, terbutaline, and theophylline	Bronchospasm and wheezing from antagonistic action of beta blocker	• Check the patient's history for asthma. • Monitor him for signs and symptoms of pulmonary disorders: wheezing, shortness of breath, restlessness, increased pulse rate, thready pulse, and dizziness. • Instruct the patient to report breathing problems and warn him not to stop taking the drug without consulting the doctor. • To minimize this interaction, the doctor may order a cardioselective beta blocker, such as atenolol or metoprolol.
• Theophylline	Reduced theophylline effectiveness from antagonistic action of beta blocker	• Monitor the patient for theophylline effectiveness. • Monitor plasma theophylline levels. Therapeutic levels range from 10 to 20 µg/ml. If necessary, suggest that the doctor increase the theophylline dosage. • Assess the patient for breathing problems. Instruct him to report breathing problems. • To minimize this interaction, the doctor may order a cardioselective beta blocker, such as atenolol or metoprolol.

metoprolol and propranolol

Interacting drug	Possible effect	Nursing considerations
• Chlorpromazine	Increased beta blocker effect from decreased first-pass metabolism of the antihypertensive	• Monitor the patient's blood pressure and pulse rate. • If necessary, suggest that the doctor decrease the beta blocker dosage.
• Barbiturates	Decreased beta blocker effectiveness from increased first-pass metabolism of barbiturates	• Monitor the patient's blood pressure and pulse rate. • If necessary, suggest that the doctor increase the beta blocker dosage.

propranolol only

Interacting drug	Possible effect	Nursing considerations
• Cimetidine	Beta blocker toxicity from inhibited metabolism or decreased first-pass effect	• Monitor the patient's blood pressure and pulse rate. • If necessary, suggest that the doctor decrease the propranolol dosage.

CONTINUED ON PAGE 110

CARDIOVASCULAR DRUGS

CARDIOVASCULAR DRUGS: INTERACTIONS AFFECTING THERAPY CONTINUED

CALCIUM CHANNEL BLOCKERS
All calcium channel blockers: diltiazem, nifedipine, verapamil

Interacting drug	Possible effect	Nursing considerations
• Beta blockers	Heart block from negative inotropic effect of both agents. *Note:* This interaction is somewhat more significant with verapamil.	• Observe the patient for signs and symptoms of congestive heart failure, such as shortness of breath and swollen ankles. Teach him to recognize and report these signs and symptoms. • Check for breathing problems and light-headedness. • Instruct the patient to count his pulse rate and to report an abnormally slow rate (less than 50 beats/minute or as specified by the doctor). • Tell him to take the drugs only in the prescribed dosages and to consult a doctor before discontinuing the drugs, taking additional medications, or drinking alcoholic beverages.
• Disopyramide	Heart block from inhibition of AV conduction by both drugs. *Note:* This interaction is somewhat more significant with verapamil.	• Follow the same guidelines listed above.
• Antihypertensives	Additive hypotension. *Note:* This interaction is somewhat more significant with nifedipine.	• Periodically check blood pressure and pulse while the patient is lying down, sitting, and standing. • Advise him to sit and stand slowly to avoid dizziness.
• Digoxin	Digitalis toxicity from increased plasma digoxin levels. *Note:* This interaction is somewhat more significant with verapamil.	• Observe the patient for signs and symptoms of digitalis toxicity: nausea and vomiting, anorexia, diarrhea, dysrhythmias, and green- or yellow-tinted vision. • Monitor plasma digoxin levels. Therapeutic levels range from 0.7 to 2.0 ng/ml. • If necessary, suggest that the doctor reduce the digoxin dosage.

DIGITALIS GLYCOSIDES
All digitalis glycosides: for example, digitalis, digitoxin, digoxin

Interacting drug	Possible effect	Nursing considerations
• Potassium-wasting diuretics; for example, thiazide diuretics and loop diuretics	Digitalis toxicity from hypokalemia	• Monitor serum potassium levels. • Check EKG readings for ST segment depression. • Observe the patient for signs and symptoms of digitalis toxicity: nausea and vomiting, anorexia, diarrhea, dysrhythmias, and green- or yellow-tinted vision.
• Thyroid hormones in very high doses	Reduced effectiveness of digitalis glycoside; mechanism unknown	• Monitor the patient for decreased response to digitalis glycoside. *Note:* A patient with a hyperthyroid condition may experience the same interaction.

digitoxin only

Interacting drug	Possible effect	Nursing consideration
• Cholestyramine - or - • Colestipol	Decreased digitoxin effect from digitoxin binding to cholestyramine or colestipol in the GI tract	• If possible, avoid this combination. • If the patient must receive this combination, increase the digitoxin dosage as ordered and monitor plasma digitoxin levels. Therapeutic levels range from 15 to 30 ng/ml.

digoxin only

Interacting drug	Possible effect	Nursing considerations
• Anticholinergics	Digoxin toxicity from increased intestinal absorption of digoxin	• Check the patient for signs and symptoms of digoxin toxicity: nausea and vomiting, anorexia, diarrhea, dysrhythmias, and green- or yellow-tinted vision.
• Metoclopramide	Decreased digoxin effect from decreased intestinal absorption of digoxin tablets	• Substitute digoxin tablets with digoxin elixir or liquid-filled capsules (Lanoxicaps*), as ordered.
• Quinidine	Digoxin toxicity from altered digoxin distribution	• Monitor plasma digoxin levels. Therapeutic levels range from 0.7 to 2 ng/ml. • Reduce the digoxin dosage, as ordered. • Check the patient for signs and symptoms of digoxin toxicity: nausea and vomiting, anorexia, diarrhea, dysrhythmias, and green- or yellow-tinted vision.

DIURETICS

All potassium-wasting diuretics: for example, thiazide diuretics and loop diuretics

Interacting drug	Possible effect	Nursing considerations
• Corticosteroids	Hypokalemia from additive effect	• Monitor serum potassium levels. • Check the patient for signs and symptoms of hypokalemia: muscle cramps, irregular heart rate, and ST segment depression on EKG.

POTASSIUM-SPARING DIURETICS

All potassium-sparing diuretics: amiloride, spironolactone, triamterene

Interacting drug	Possible effect	Nursing considerations
• Potassium supplements	Hyperkalemia from potassium retention	• Monitor serum potassium levels. • Check EKG readings for widening of QRS complexes, tall T waves, and ventricular fibrillation. • Observe the patient for other signs and symptoms of hyperkalemia: muscular weakness, paralysis, and abdominal cramps. • Instruct the patient to minimize intake of foods high in potassium (such as fruits and leafy green vegetables) and to avoid drastic dietary changes.

spironolactone only

Interacting drug	Possible effect	Nursing considerations
• Aspirin	Reduced diuretic effect from negation of renal action of spironolactone	• Tell the patient to avoid over-the-counter products containing aspirin. • Monitor his condition for diuretic effectiveness.

*Not available in Canada

G.I. DRUGS

G.I. DRUGS: INTERACTIONS AFFECTING THERAPY

Like analgesics, most antacids are readily available as over-the-counter products. But, of course, just because a drug is available without a prescription doesn't mean it's harmless. When a patient takes an antacid, the medication alters gastric pH. And because pH balance plays such an important role in absorption of orally administered drugs, the antacid can set the stage for a variety of drug interactions.

Antacids may also physically bind with certain other drugs, reducing or preventing their absorption. As you learned on page 96, you shouldn't give an antacid containing calcium, magnesium, or aluminum to a patient taking tetracycline. By binding with tetracycline, the antacid inhibits absorption, limiting the antibiotic effect.

Enteric-coated drugs shouldn't be given concurrently with antacids either; the antacid can destroy the coating. This means that instead of being absorbed in the small intestine—the intended destination—the enteric-coated drug is absorbed directly by the gastric mucosa, possibly causing nausea, vomiting, and stomach irritation.

Cimetidine, a popular antiulcer drug, doesn't seem to affect drug absorption. But it can slow drug metabolism and prolong the duration of action of other drugs. Be especially alert for signs and symptoms of excessive sedation in the patient who's taking cimetidine along with some benzodiazepines, such as diazepam.

ALL ANTACIDS

Interacting drug	Possible effect	Nursing consideration
• All enteric-coated products, including some forms of aspirin; for example, Ecotrin	Premature drug dissolution in the stomach; antacids destroy enteric coating	• Administer drugs 1 hour apart.

ANTACIDS CONTAINING CALCIUM, MAGNESIUM, OR ALUMINUM
For example: Di-Gel*, Maalox Plus, Mylanta

Interacting drug	Possible effect	Nursing considerations
• Iron salts	• Decreased iron absorption from iron precipitation, causing decreased response in treating anemia	• Administer drugs 2 hours apart. • Monitor the patient for decreased hematologic response to iron salt therapy.

CIMETIDINE

Interacting drug	Possible effect	Nursing considerations
• All benzodiazepines (except lorazepam, oxazepam, and temazepam)	Excessive sedation from decreased metabolism of benzodiazepines	• Decrease benzodiazepine dosage, as ordered. • Check the patient for unusual fatigue. • Instruct the patient to take the drugs exactly as prescribed and to notify the doctor before adding other medications, alcoholic beverages, or over-the-counter products containing alcohol. Warn him that this combination may cause drowsiness. • Tell him to notify the doctor if he experiences slurred speech, unsteady gait, or extreme fatigue.
• Theophylline	Theophylline toxicity from decreased theophylline metabolism	• Monitor plasma theophylline levels. Therapeutic levels range from 10 to 20 µg/ml. • Check the patient for signs and symptoms of theophylline toxicity: anorexia, nausea and vomiting, headache, tachycardia, dizziness, and restlessness.

*Not available in Canada

HORMONES

HORMONES: INTERACTIONS AFFECTING THERAPY

You've probably seen it happen more than once: the stiff, swollen joints of a patient with rheumatoid arthritis responding to prednisone treatment within a few days; or the patient with severe hay fever getting quick relief from an injection of methylprednisolone (Medrol). But, like all corticosteroids, these drugs can profoundly alter the body's metabolism and immune responses. As a result, when other medications are added to the patient's drug therapy, the chances of an adverse reaction from a drug interaction increase.

Keep in mind that corticosteroids can make a patient susceptible to hypokalemia. If your patient's receiving a thiazide or loop diuretic while on corticosteroid therapy, be sure to continuously monitor serum potassium levels and check EKG readings periodically. *Caution:* If your patient is taking a digitalis glycoside, monitor him carefully for signs and symptoms of digitalis toxicity. Hypokalemia predisposes him to this adverse reaction.

If your female patient's receiving barbiturates or rifampin while taking an oral contraceptive, urge her to use an additional birth control method. Why? Rifampin and barbiturates can increase the metabolism of an oral contraceptive, making it less effective.

CORTICOSTEROIDS
All corticosteroids: for example, cortisone, dexamethasone, methylprednisolone, prednisone

Interacting drug	Possible effect	Nursing considerations
• Nonsteroidal anti-inflammatory drugs; for example, fenoprofen and ibuprofen - or - • Salicylates	GI ulcers from additive GI irritation	• Administer with food, milk, or antacids. • Assess the patient for developing ulcers. Keep in mind that the anti-inflammatory drug may mask pain and other ulcer symptoms.
• Digitalis glycosides	Digitalis toxicity from hypokalemia caused by corticosteroids	• Monitor serum potassium levels. Normal levels range from 3.8 to 5.0 mEq/liter. • Observe the patient for signs and symptoms of digitalis toxicity: anorexia, nausea and vomiting, diarrhea, mental depression, dysrhythmias, and yellow- or green-tinted vision. • Regularly monitor pulse rate, rhythm, and quality. • Encourage the patient to eat foods high in potassium, such as fruits and leafy green vegetables.
• Barbiturates - or - • Phenytoin - or - • Rifampin	Decreased corticosteroid effect from increased hepatic metabolism of corticosteroids	• Monitor corticosteroid effectiveness. If necessary, suggest that the doctor increase corticosteroid dosage.
• All potassium-wasting diuretics, especially thiazides and loop diuretics - or - • Amphotericin B	Hypokalemia from additive effects	• Monitor serum potassium levels. Normal levels range from 3.8 to 5.0 mEq/liter. • Periodically monitor the patient's EKG readings for signs of hypokalemia; for example, flat or inverted T waves, depressed ST segments, and widening of QRS complexes. • Encourage the patient to eat foods high in potassium, such as fruits and leafy green vetetables.

CONTINUED ON PAGE 114

IDENTIFYING DRUG INTERACTIONS

HORMONES

HORMONES: INTERACTIONS AFFECTING THERAPY CONTINUED

ORAL CONTRACEPTIVES

Interacting drug	Possible effect	Nursing considerations
• Barbiturates - or - • Rifampin	Reduced contraceptive effectiveness from increased metabolism of oral contraceptive	• Advise the patient to use an additional birth control method while taking barbiturates or rifampin; or ask the doctor to substitute one of the drugs with a non-interacting one.
• Theophylline	Increased risk of theophylline toxicity because theophylline metabolism is inhibited by oral contraceptives	• Monitor plasma theophylline levels. Therapeutic levels range from 10 to 20 µg/ml. • Check the patient for signs and symptoms of theophylline toxicity: anorexia, nausea and vomiting, headache, tachycardia, dizziness, and restlessness.

THYROID HORMONES
All thyroid hormones: levothyroxine, liothyronine, liotrix, thyroglobulin, thyroid

Interacting drug	Possible effect	Nursing consideration
• Cholestyramine - or - • Colestipol	Decreased thyroid hormone effectiveness from decreased intestinal absorption of thyroid hormones	• Administer cholestyramine and colestipol at least 4 hours before or after a thyroid hormone.

THYROID HORMONE ANTAGONISTS
methimazole and propylthiouracil

Interacting drug	Possible effect	Nursing considerations
• Digitalis glycosides	Digitalis toxicity; mechanism unknown	• Monitor the patient for signs and symptoms of digitalis toxicity: anorexia, nausea and vomiting, diarrhea, mental depression, dysrhythmias, and yellow- or green-tinted vision. • Regularly monitor his pulse rate, rhythm, and quality. • Monitor plasma digitalis levels. Reduce the digitalis dosage, if ordered.

PSYCHOTHERAPEUTIC DRUGS

PSYCHOTHERAPEUTIC DRUGS: INTERACTIONS AFFECTING THERAPY

Psychotherapeutic drugs can treat a wide range of conditions, including psychosis, anxiety, and depression. Read what follows to learn about special considerations for drugs in this category.

Tricyclic antidepressants (TCAs) have an anticholinergic effect. So, if you're administering a TCA with another anticholinergic drug (such as belladonna or propantheline), monitor your patient for blurred vision, drowsiness, constipation, urinary retention, and other signs and symptoms of excessive anticholinergic response. *Important:* Check you patient's history for problems that may be exacerbated by enhanced anticholinergic effects; for example, glaucoma and bladder neck obstruction.

Avoid administering a TCA to a patient who's receiving the antihypertensive agents guanethidine or clonidine. Such a combination usually results in poor hypertension control.

Chances are you'll rarely have to administer a *monoamine oxidase (MAO) inhibitor*, since doctors seldom prescribe these drugs for depression anymore. Nevertheless, don't forget that MAO inhibitors can cause serious adverse reactions when combined with certain other medications. Interactions with sympathomimetic drugs, TCAs, and meperidine can lead to serious cardiovascular problems, such as hypertension or hypotension.

If you're administering an MAO inhibitor with a TCA, closely monitor your patient for toxic effects of both drugs, in addition to signs and symptoms of cardiovascular problems.

And warn the patient using an MAO inhibitor to avoid foods high in tyramine, which is normally destroyed by the MAO enzyme. When the MAO enzyme is inhibited, tyramine isn't broken down. Tyramine then causes norepinephrine to be released from adrenergic nerve endings, which could cause hypertensive crisis. Foods high in tyramine include liver, sherry, chocolate, Chianti wine, pickled herring, and aged cheeses. Instruct the patient to wait 2 to 3 weeks after discontinuing the MAO inhibitor before eating foods that contain tyramine.

Barbiturates speed the metabolism of many drugs. So, oral anticoagulants, beta blockers, corticosteroids, doxycycline, oral contraceptives, and quinidine may not be as effective when combined with a barbiturate.

If you've ever cared for a patient who received a *phenothiazine*, you may have discovered that interactions with anticholinergic agents and antacids curbed the phenothiazine's antipsychotic effect. And, like TCAs, phenothiazines can also interfere with guanethidine's antihypertensive effects.

Lithium can be toxic when given with indomethacin or a thiazide or loop diuretic. Stay alert for such adverse reactions as central nervous system depression, tremors, GI irritation, dizziness, headache, confusion, and mental dullness. Also monitor plasma lithium levels, as ordered.

TRICYCLIC ANTIDEPRESSANTS (TCAs)

All tricyclic antidepressants: for example, amitriptyline, amoxapine, desipramine, doxepin, imipramine, maprotiline, nortriptyline, protriptyline, trimipramine

Interacting drug	Possible effect	Nursing considerations
• Epinephrine - or - • Norepinephrine	Increased sympathomimetic effect from drug synergism	• Decrease the dosage of these sympathomimetic drugs, if ordered. • Check the patient's history for cardiac problems. • Monitor for increased sympathomimetic effects, such as increased heart rate. • Monitor blood pressure and pulse; report deviations from baseline.
• MAO inhibitors	Enhanced effect or toxicity of either drug; mechanism unknown	• Use this combination with extreme caution. • Immediately report indications of toxicity from either drug (for example, nausea, dizziness, convulsions, and seizures). Stop one or both drugs, as ordered.

CONTINUED ON PAGE 116

IDENTIFYING DRUG INTERACTIONS

PSYCHOTHERAPEUTIC DRUGS

PSYCHOTHERAPEUTIC DRUGS: INTERACTIONS AFFECTING THERAPY CONTINUED

TRICYCLIC ANTIDEPRESSANTS (TCAs) continued

All tricyclic antidepressants: for example, amitriptyline, amoxapine, desipramine, doxepin, imipramine, maprotiline, nortriptyline, protriptyline, trimipramine

Interacting drug	Possible effect	Nursing considerations
• Gastrointestinal anticholinergics; for example, propantheline and belladonna	Dry mouth and eyes, blurred vision, tachycardia, constipation, urinary retention, drowsiness, and disorientation from additive anticholinergic effect	• Monitor the patient for increased heart rate and vision changes. • Check his history for glaucoma, urinary retention, and prostate disorders. • Monitor his fluid intake and urinary output for excessive urine retention. • Modify his diet and encourage adequate fluid intake to avoid constipation. • Suggest that he suck on ice chips or hard candy to relieve dry mouth. • Warn him to notify the doctor if he becomes overheated easily or if his eyes become sensitive to light. Both symptoms indicate toxicity. • Advise him to use caution when operating machinery or driving because he may feel drowsy.

BARBITURATES

All barbiturates: for example, amobarbital, butabarbital, pentobarbital, phenobarbital, secobarbital

Interacting drug	Possible effect	Nursing considerations
• Beta adrenergic blockers; for example, propranolol and metoprolol	Decreased beta adrenergic blocker effectiveness from increase in first-pass metabolism	• Monitor the patient for reduced effectiveness of beta adrenergic blocker. Consider the beta blocker to be effective if your patient's pulse rate doesn't increase after a position change from sitting to standing. • If necessary, increase the beta blocker dosage, as ordered.
• Corticosteroids - or - • Doxycycline - or - • Oral contraceptives - or - • Quinidine	Decreased effectiveness of the interacting drug from increased metabolism	• Increase dosage of the interacting drug, if ordered. • Monitor the patient for decreased therapeutic effect. • If the patient's using an oral contraceptive while receiving barbiturates, advise her to use an additional birth control method. • If the patient's receiving quinidine with barbiturates, monitor plasma quinidine levels and check his EKG frequently.
• Alcohol	Additive and synergistic CNS and respiratory depression; possibly fatal	• Warn the patient to avoid alcohol, including over-the-counter drugs containing alcohol (for example, liquid cough and cold preparations).

PHENOTHIAZINES AND HALOPERIDOL

All phenothiazines: for example, chlorpromazine, prochlorperazine, promazine, thioridazine

Interacting drug	Possible effect	Nursing considerations
• Antacids	Reduced antipsychotic effect from decreased absorption of phenothiazine	• Administer these drugs 2 hours apart. • Observe the patient for worsened psychotic state.
• Anticholinergics; for example, atropine, benztropine, scopolamine	Decreased antipsychotic effect from drug antagonism; increased adverse anticholinergic effects	• Monitor the patient for reduced phenothiazine or haloperidol effect. • Increase phenothiazine or haloperidol dosage, if ordered. This drug combination can be used safely if the dosage is carefully titrated according to the patient's response.
• Alcohol	Increase in adverse effects of both drugs from additive or synergistic CNS effects	• Monitor the patient for excessive sedation and impaired psychomotor function. • Advise him to avoid driving and other activities requiring alertness.

LITHIUM

Interacting drug	Possible effect	Nursing considerations
• All potassium-losing diuretics (thiazides and loop diuretics) - or - • Indomethacin	Lithium toxicity from decreased lithium excretion	• Monitor plasma lithium levels. Toxic levels are above 1.5 mEq/liter. • Monitor the patient for signs and symptoms of lithium toxicity: nausea, vomiting, and other symptoms of GI irritation; fluid retention (indicated by edema and weight gain); dizziness; headache; tremors; and mental dullness. • Warn the patient not to take any over-the-counter drugs (especially diuretics) unless the doctor or pharmacist approves. • Before discharge, teach him to recognize signs and symptoms of lithium toxicity, including sudden weight gain, bloated face or ankles, extreme fatigue or weakness, slurred speech, or jerking of arms or legs.
• Methyldopa	Lithium toxicity from altered lithium distribution	• Monitor plasma lithium levels. Toxic levels are above 1.5 mEq/liter. • Regularly assess the patient for adverse CNS effects: mental confusion, slurred speech, drowsiness, and blurred vision. • Monitor the patient for signs and symptoms of lithium toxicity: nausea, vomiting, and other symptoms of GI irritation; fluid retention (indicated by edema and weight gain); dizziness; headache; tremors; and mental dullness. • Before discharge, teach him to recognize signs and symptoms of lithium toxicity, including sudden weight gain, bloated face or ankles, extreme fatigue or weakness, slurred speech, or jerking of arms or legs.

CONTINUED ON PAGE 118

PSYCHOTHERAPEUTIC DRUGS

PSYCHOTHERAPEUTIC DRUGS: INTERACTIONS AFFECTING THERAPY CONTINUED

LITHIUM continued

Interacting drug	Possible effect	Nursing considerations
• Urinary alkalinizers; for example, antacids, carbonic anhydrase inhibitors	Decreased lithium effectiveness from hastened renal excretion of lithium	• Monitor plasma lithium levels and therapeutic response. • Observe the patient for worsening of his psychiatric condition. • Increase lithium dosage, if ordered.

MONOAMINE OXIDASE (MAO) INHIBITORS
All MAO inhibitors: for example, isocarboxazid, phenelzine, procarbazine, tranylcypromine

Interacting drug	Possible effect	Nursing considerations
• Sympathomimetics; for example, amphetamines, norepinephrine, metaproterenol, and pseudoephedrine	Hypertension and other serious cardiovascular disorders from excessive catecholamine release	• Don't administer these drugs together. • Advise the patient not to use over-the-counter preparations containing sympathomimetic drugs, such as diet pills, cold and allergy medicines, and nasal sprays. Tell him to check with the pharmacist before buying over-the-counter drugs.
• Tricyclic antidepressants	Hypertension and other serious cardiovascular disorders; mechanism unknown	• Use this drug combination with caution. • Monitor the patient's blood pressure and heart rate.
• Levodopa	Levodopa toxicity from reduced levodopa metabolism	• Monitor the patient for signs and symptoms of levodopa toxicity, such as flushing, hypertension, and tachycardia. • Reduce levodopa dosage, if ordered. • Keep phentolamine available in case hypertension occurs.
• Insulin	Increased effect of insulin, possibly causing hypoglycemia; mechanism unknown	• Monitor the patient's serum glucose levels and dietary intake. Adjust insulin dosage, as ordered.

MISCELLANEOUS DRUGS

OTHER DRUG INTERACTIONS AFFECTING THERAPY

VITAMIN B_6

Interacting drug	Possible effect	Nursing consideration
• Levodopa	Decreased antiparkinson effectiveness of levodopa from increased levodopa metabolism	• Avoid administering vitamin B_6 to a patient who's receiving levodopa; or ask the doctor to substitute levodopa with levodopa-carbidopa (Sinemet) to avoid this interaction.

FOLIC ACID

Interacting drug	Possible effect	Nursing consideration
• Sulfasalazine	Reduced folic acid effectiveness from decreased GI absorption of folic acid	• If folic acid replacement is required, make sure the doctor orders a parenteral route.

KETAMINE

Interacting drug	Possible effect	Nursing considerations
• Halothane	Decreased cardiac function and hypotension from antagonistic action of halothane that blocks cardiovascular stimulation by ketamine	• Monitor the patient's cardiac output; pulse, rhythm, rate, and quality; and blood pressure.
• Tubocurarine	Prolonged respiratory depression; mechanism unknown	• Use this combination cautiously. • Monitor the patient's respiratory rate. • Provide mechanical respiratory support.

VITAMIN B_{12}

Interacting drug	Possible effect	Nursing considerations
• Para-aminosalicylic acid	Reduced vitamin B_{12} effectiveness from decreased GI absorption of vitamin B_{12}	• Administer vitamin B_{12} by a parenteral route, as ordered.
• Chloramphenicol	Decreased effectiveness of vitamin B_{12} in treatment of anemia from chloramphenicol-induced inhibition of hemoglobin synthesis	• Be aware that the patient's response to vitamin B_{12} therapy may be delayed. • Monitor the patient's complete blood cell count, as ordered.

LAB TESTS

HOW DRUGS AFFECT TEST RESULTS

Like most nurses, you probably spend part of the day evaluating laboratory test results. But do you know that many drugs can alter test values, possibly causing incorrect findings that could lead to the wrong diagnosis?

When you consider the fact that some hospitalized patients receive eight or more medications concurrently, you can see why you must consider your patient's drug therapy when reviewing his laboratory test findings. Read what follows for some important points to keep in mind.

Methodologic effects. A drug can affect the outcome of a laboratory test in one of two ways. The first, known as a *methodologic* effect, occurs when a drug interferes with testing methods. The result is an incorrect value—a false increase, false decrease, or false-normal value for the body function or fluid being measured.

As an example, consider the serum bilirubin test, which is based on serum color. If your patient has received a drug that gives serum a yellowish cast, laboratory test values may incorrectly indicate an elevated bilirubin level. Even ascorbic acid (vitamin C) can have this effect, so don't forget to ask about vitamin supplements when taking a drug history.

To learn which drugs can produce false values in laboratory tests, refer to the chart on the following page.

Pharmacologic effects. The second type of effect is *pharmacologic*, which means that the drug actually alters the level of the body fluid constituent being measured, either through the drug's normal pharmacologic properties or through a toxic reaction. The resulting test value, although accurate, is misleading unless the drug's effect is taken into account.

The urine phenolsulfonphthalein (PSP) test, a kidney function study, provides an example of this type of drug effect. The PSP test, as you know, measures renal tubular secretion. Many drugs, including salicylates, sulfonamides, and penicillins, can inhibit tubular secretion, causing an actual, or *true*, decrease in urine PSP levels.

Remember, some drugs can alter test values for several weeks after the drug has been discontinued. Keep this in mind if you come across a surprising laboratory finding after drug therapy has been stopped or changed.

Some drugs can have toxic effects on an organ. For instance, novobiocin, rifampin, and I.V. fat emulsions can cause liver toxicity. So before concluding, strictly on the basis of liver function studies, that your patient has liver disease, first review his drug history closely for use of a potentially hepatotoxic drug.

Beginning on page 122, you'll find a chart of drugs that can alter test measurements pharmacologically. But this chart doesn't include drugs that have an *intended* pharmacologic effect on the function or body fluid being measured. Warfarin, for instance, is expected to increase prothrombin time, so it doesn't appear in this chart.

Some pharmacologic effects call for special nursing measures. Find out about these by reading the nursing considerations for each test.

Your role. By providing a vital communication link between the doctor and laboratory personnel, you're in a unique position to prevent misinterpretation of laboratory test results. Chances are, the doctor doesn't know the intricacies of testing procedures or which drugs can interfere with the tests he's ordered. Laboratory personnel, on the other hand, have this information but don't know which drugs the patient's receiving.

Where do you come in? On the laboratory slip sent along with the specimen, list all the drugs your patient's receiving that may interfere with test results. (For guidelines, consult the following charts and your hospital's laboratory manual.) The laboratory technician often can tailor his test methods to the patient's drug therapy, reducing the chance of a drug-induced alteration.

Also, learn about drug interactions and testing procedures, so you can anticipate a misleading laboratory finding or suggest that a test value be disregarded if you suspect drug interference has occurred.

What should you do if laboratory findings don't correlate well with the doctor's diagnosis or your clinical assessment of a patient? Suggest that the test be repeated using a different procedure that adjusts for or eliminates drug interference.

But remember—even if you know a drug *can* alter laboratory test results, you can't be certain that it *will* in every case. That's why the doctor may order a particular test even if he knows your patient's receiving a drug that may alter test results. In some cases, of course, he may withhold a drug to minimize the possibility of a misleading test value.

METHODOLOGIC INTERACTIONS

Some laboratory tests yield false-positive or false-negative results after administration of certain drugs. For details, read this chart.

SERUM BILIRUBIN

These drugs can cause a false increase:
- ascorbic acid
- dextran
- I.V. fat emulsion*

This drug can cause a false decrease:
- ascorbic acid

PLASMA CORTISOL

These drugs can cause a false increase:
- estrogen*
- heparin
- spironolactone

SERUM GLUCOSE

This drug can cause a false increase:
- dextran

This drug can cause a false decrease:
- acetaminophen

SERUM MAGNESIUM

This drug can cause a false decrease:
- calcium gluconate

BROMSULPHALEIN (BSP)

These drugs can cause a false increase:
- heparin
- phenazopyridine
- phenolphthalein

THYROID FUNCTION

These drugs can cause a false increase in protein-bound iodine (PBI):
- barium sulfate
- inorganic iodides (especially potassium iodide)
- iodine-containing contrast media*
- isopropamide

* May also have a pharmacologic effect. See the chart beginning on page 122.

SERUM URIC ACID

These drugs can cause a false increase:
- aminophylline
- ascorbic acid
- levodopa

Note: Coffee consumption may cause the same effect.

URINE CATECHOLAMINES

These drugs can cause a false increase:
- chloral hydrate
- erythromycin
- methyldopa*
- phenothiazines
- quinidine
- quinine
- tetracyclines
- vitamin B complex

URINE 5-HYDROXYINDOLEACETIC ACID (5-HIAA)

These drugs can cause a false increase:
- acetaminophen
- guaifenesin
- methocarbamol
- salicylates

These drugs can cause a false decrease:
- methenamine
- phenothiazines

URINE KETONES

These drugs can cause a false positive:
- captopril
- levodopa
- phenazopyridine
- phenothiazines
- salicylates
- valproic acid

URINE PHENOLSULFONPHTHALEIN (PSP)

These drugs can cause a false positive:
- cascara

- danthron
- phenazopyridine
- phenolphthalein

URINE PROTEIN

These drugs can cause a false positive:
- acetazolamide
- aminosalicylic acid
- cephalosporins
- iodine-containing contrast media*
- levodopa
- penicillins (in very large doses)
- phenazopyridine
- sodium bicarbonate
- sulfonamides
- tolbutamide
- tolmetin

URINE STEROIDS

These drugs can cause a false increase in 17-ketogenic steroids, 17-ketosteroids, or 17-hydroxycorticosteroids:
- cephalosporins
- digitalis glycosides
- ethinamate
- hydralazine
- meprobamate
- methenamine
- nalidixic acid
- naproxen
- penicillin G
- phenothiazines

These drugs can cause a false decrease in one or more urine steroids:
- calcium gluconate
- carbamazepine
- reserpine

URINE VANILLYLMANDELIC ACID (VMA)

These drugs can cause a false increase:
- methocarbamol
- phenolsulfonphthalein
- salicylates

These drugs can cause a false decrease:
- levodopa
- salicylates

LAB TESTS

PHARMACOLOGIC INTERACTIONS

Some laboratory test results are misleading because they reflect alterations caused by a drug's usual pharmacologic effects or by a toxic effect. Read the following chart to learn more.

SERUM BILIRUBIN

Drug	Possible effect	Nursing considerations
• iopanoic acid	true but transient increase	• Monitor the patient's liver function studies.
• I.V. fat emulsion*	true increase from liver toxicity	• Check his history for indications of liver disorders, including alcoholism.
• novobiocin	true increase from liver toxicity	• Observe him for jaundice and other signs and symptoms of a liver disorder.
• rifampin	true but transient increase from liver toxicity	

PLASMA CORTISOL

Drug	Possible effect	Nursing consideration
• amphetamines	true increase, especially when drug is given I.V. and when the laboratory test is performed in the morning	• When taking a patient history, be sure to ask about smoking and consumption of alcoholic beverages.
• ethanol	true increase in most patients; true decrease in alcoholic patients	
• nicotine	true increase	
• vasopressin	true increase	

SERUM GAMMA GLUTAMYL TRANSPEPTIDASE (GGT)

Drug	Possible effect	Nursing considerations
• barbiturates	true but transient increase	• Monitor the patient's liver function studies, as ordered.
• clofibrate	true decrease	• Check for signs and symptoms of a liver disorder.
• ethanol	true increase, which may persist for several days after a single dose	
• streptokinase	true but transient increase	

SERUM GLUCOSE

Drug	Possible effect	Nursing considerations
• acetazolamide	true increase in diabetic patients	• Monitor serum glucose levels closely, as ordered.
• beta blockers	true decrease from blockage of normal glycogen release after hypoglycemia	• Monitor the patient for signs and symptoms of hypoglycemia and hyperglycemia.
• corticosteroids	true increase, especially in diabetic patients, following topical, oral, or parenteral administration	• Check his urine for sugar and acetone.
• diazoxide	true increase, probably from impaired insulin release	• Check his diet for foods that could alter serum glucose levels. Specifically note the types and amount of food he's eaten during the day.
• diuretics	true increase, especially in diabetics, from impaired glucose tolerance	
• epinephrine	true increase from release of glycogen stores from the liver	
• estrogens	true increase, especially in high doses, from impaired glucose tolerance	
• ethanol	true decrease	
• salicylates	true decrease in diabetics; true increase or decrease in patients with overdose	

*May also have a methodologic effect. See the chart on page 121.

IDENTIFYING DRUG INTERACTIONS

SERUM PROLACTIN

Drug	Possible effect	Nursing consideration
• ergot alkaloids (for example, bromocriptine, ergonovine, and ergotamine)	true decrease, especially in patients with initially high serum prolactin values	• Methyldopa may raise serum prolactin sufficiently to cause lactation in females.
• levodopa	true decrease even after a single dose, especially in patients with initially high serum prolactin values	
• MAO inhibitors	true increase only with long-term therapy	
• methyldopa	true increase	
• metoclopramide	true increase from stimulation of prolactin secretion	
• oral contraceptives	true increase	
• phenothiazines, haloperidol, and thiothixene	true increase, even after a single dose, from dopaminergic blockade; more likely with long-term therapy	

THYROID FUNCTION

Drug	Possible effect	Nursing consideration
• estrogen	true increase in thyroxine-binding globulin (TBG) and thyroxine (T_4), which may persist for several weeks after medication is discontinued	• Monitor the patient for signs and symptoms of hypothyroidism and hyperthyroidism.
• lithium	true decrease in T_4	
• methadone	true increase in T_4, triiodothyronine (T_3) uptake, and TBG; true decrease in resin T_3	
• para-aminosalicylic acid	true decrease in T_4 and protein-bound iodine (PBI)	
• phenytoin	true decrease in T_4 and T_3 uptake	

SERUM URIC ACID

Drug	Possible effect	Nursing considerations
• diazoxide	true increase, when given in large doses, from decreased uric acid excretion	• Ask the patient if he has a history of gout or if anyone in his family has gout. • Check the patient for signs and symptoms of gout; for example, swelling and pain in the joints. • Increased serum uric acid levels may require treatment with allopurinol or uricosuric drugs, such as probenecid.
• diuretics (thiazides, thiazide-like diuretics, and such loop diuretics as ethacrynic acid and furosemide)	true increase from inhibited tubular secretion of uric acid	

CONTINUED ON PAGE 124

LAB TESTS

PHARMACOLOGIC INTERACTIONS CONTINUED

SERUM URIC ACID continued

Drug	Possible effect	Nursing considerations
• ethambutol	true increase, when given in large doses, from altered renal uric acid clearance	• Ask the patient if he has a history of gout or if anyone in his family has gout. • Check the patient for signs and symptoms of gout; for example, swelling and pain in the joints. • Increased serum uric acid levels may require treatment with allopurinol or uricosuric drugs, such as probenecid.
• methotrexate	true increase from cell destruction, causing uric acid release	
• pyrazinamide	true increase, when given in large doses, from inhibited uric acid excretion	
• salicylates	true decrease when given in large doses; true increase when given in small doses	

URINE CATECHOLAMINES

Drug	Possible effect	Nursing considerations
• aminophylline	true increase in epinephrine and norepinephrine levels	• As ordered, withhold these drugs several days prior to test (especially methyldopa). • Monitor the patient for blood pressure changes if methyldopa is being withheld.
• caffeine	true increase in epinephrine and norepinephrine levels	
• clonidine	true decrease during drug therapy; true increase when drug is discontinued	
• epinephrine	true increase in epinephrine levels, especially when drug is given in high doses and when administered subcutaneously	
• insulin	true increase in epinephrine levels	
• isoproterenol	true increase in epinephrine and norepinephrine levels	
• methyldopa*	true increase	

URINE PROTEIN

Drug	Possible effect	Nursing consideration
• iodine-containing contrast media* and other nephrotoxic drugs (for example, aminoglycosides)	true increase from kidney toxicity	• Monitor kidney function studies, as ordered: creatinine and blood urea nitrogen.

URINE STEROIDS

Drug	Possible effect	Nursing consideration
• aminoglutethimide	true decrease in 17-hydroxycorticosteroids, 17-ketogenic steroids, and 17-ketosteroids	• Levels increase with severe physical and emotional stress.
• androgens	true increase in 17-hydroxycorticosteroids, 17-ketogenic steroids and 17-ketosteroids	
• corticosteroids	true decrease in 17-hydroxycorticosteroids and 17-ketosteroids	
• iodine-containing contrast media	true decrease in 17-ketogenic steroids	

*May also have a methodologic effect. See the chart on page 121.

URINE STEROIDS

Drug	Possible effect	Nursing consideration
• mitotane	true decrease in 17-hydroxycorticosteroids	• Levels increase with severe physical and emotional stress.
• oral contraceptives	true decrease in 17-hydroxycorticosteroids, 17-ketogenic steroids, and 17-ketosteroids	
• probenecid	true decrease in 17-ketosteroids	
• testolactone	true increase in 17-ketosteroids	

URINE VANILLYLMANDELIC ACID (VMA)

Drug	Possible effect	Nursing consideration
• bretylium	true decrease	• Monitor the patient for increased or decreased blood pressure.
• epinephrine	true increase	
• levodopa*	true increase	
• nitroglycerin	true increase	

*May also have a methodologic effect. See the chart on page 121.

DRUGS THAT ALTER URINE COLOR

Drug	Urine Color Change
ferrous salts iron sorbitex quinine	black
methylene blue triamterene (causes a pale blue color)	blue
amitriptyline methylene blue	blue-green
chloroquine furazolidone methocarbamol metronidazole nitrofurantoin primaquine quinine sulfonamides	brown
indomethacin resorcinol	green
chlorzoxazone ethoxazene fluorescein phenazopyridine phenindione (in alkaline urine)	orange

Drug	Urine Color Change
rifampin sulfasalazine warfarin	orange
cascara (in alkaline urine) danthron phenindione phenolphthalein (in alkaline urine) phenothiazines phensuximide phenytoin senna (in alkaline urine)	pink
anthraquinone laxative (in alkaline urine) danthron daunorubicin deferoxamine ethoxazene phenazopyridine phenolphthalein (in alkaline urine) phensuximide phenytoin rifampin	red

Drug	Urine Color Change
phenazopyridine phenindione phenothiazines phensuximide phenytoin primaquine	red-brown
quinacrine riboflavin	yellow
cascara (in acid urine) chloroquine furazolidone levodopa methyldopa nitrofurantoin phenolphthalein (in acid urine) primaquine senna (in acid urine)	yellow-brown
levodopa methocarbamol methyldopa	dark urine (when urine is left standing)

APPENDIX

I.V. SOLUTION COMPATIBILITIES

Use this chart as a guide to I.V. solution compatibilities. But keep in mind that physical compatibility does not exclude the possibility of therapeutic incompatibility.

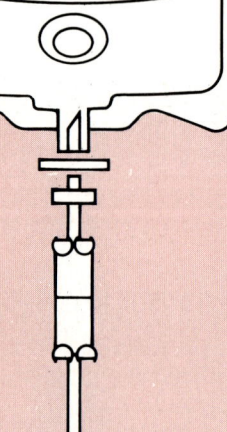

Key:
C = Compatible
I = Incompatible
O = Data unavailable
2, 4, 8, 24 = Compatible only for the number of hours indicated
X = Identical drug

	albumin	amikacin	aminophylline	amino acid injection	ampicillin	bretylium	calcium gluconate	carbenicillin	cefamandole	cefazolin	cefoxitin	cephalothin	chloramphenicol	cimetidine	clindamycin	corticotropin (ACTH)
albumin	X	O	O	O	O	O	O	O	O	O	O	O	O	O	O	O
amikacin	O	X	8	O	I	O	24	8	I	8	I	I	24	24	24	O
aminophylline	O	8	X	24	I	O	C	C	O	O	O	I	O	I	I	I
amino acid injection	O	O	24	X	12	O	24	24	O	24	O	24	1	24	24	O
ampicillin	O	I	I	I	X	O	I	I	O	O	O	O	1	C	I	O
bretylium	O	O	O	O	O	X	O	O	O	O	O	O	O	O	O	O
calcium gluconate	O	24	C	24	I	O	X	C	I	I	O	I	C	O	I	O
carbenicillin	O	8	C	24	I	O	C	X	O	C	O	O	I	O	24	O
cefamandole	O	I	O	O	O	O	I	O	X	O	O	O	O	O	O	O
cefazolin	O	8	O	24	O	I	C	O	O	X	O	O	24	24	24	O
cefoxitin	O	I	O	O	O	O	O	O	O	O	X	O	O	O	O	O
cephalothin	O	I	I	24	O	O	I	O	O	O	O	X	C	24	24	O
chloramphenicol	O	24	O	O	1	O	C	I	O	24	O	C	X	O	O	O
cimetidine	O	24	I	24	C	O	I	O	O	24	O	24	O	X	24	24
clindamycin	O	24	I	24	O	O	O	24	O	O	O	24	O	24	X	O
corticotropin (ACTH)	O	O	I	O	I	O	O	O	O	O	O	O	C	O	O	X
dexamethasone	O	I	O	O	O	O	O	O	O	O	O	O	O	O	O	O
dextrose 5% in water	C	24	C	C	2	C	C	C	C	C	C	C	C	C	C	C
dextrose 5% in lactated Ringer's	C	24	C	C	4	C	C	C	C	C	C	C	C	C	C	C
dextrose 5% in 0.45% NaCl	C	24	C	C	4	C	C	C	C	C	C	C	C	C	C	C
dextrose 5% in 0.9% NaCl	C	24	C	C	4	C	C	C	C	C	C	C	C	C	C	C
diphenhydramine	O	24	C	O	O	O	O	O	O	O	O	I	C	O	O	O
dobutamine	O	O	O	O	O	O	I	O	O	O	O	O	O	O	O	O
dopamine	O	O	I	24	I	C	24	24	O	O	O	6	24	O	O	O
epinephrine	O	24	I	O	O	O	I	I	O	O	O	I	I	O	O	O
erythromycin (I.V.) lactobionate	O	I	C	24	O	O	C	I	O	I	O	I	I	O	C	O
gentamicin	O	I	I	24	O	I	O	I	I	I	I	I	I	24	24	I
heparin sodium	O	I	C	24	I	O	C	O	O	O	O	8	C	O	24	24
hydrocortisone Na succinate	O	O	C	O	C	O	C	24	O	O	O	24	C	O	24	24
insulin (regular)	O	O	I	24	O	O	O	O	O	O	O	8	O	24	O	O
isoproterenol	O	O	I	O	O	O	O	O	O	O	O	C	O	O	O	O
kanamycin	O	O	C	C	I	O	I	I	O	I	24	I	C	O	24	O
lactated Ringer's	C	O	C	C	8	C	C	C	C	C	C	C	C	C	C	C
lidocaine	O	O	C	24	I	C	C	C	C	O	O	I	C	O	O	O
metaraminol	O	24	C	24	I	O	O	O	O	O	O	C	C	O	O	O
methicillin	O	I	C	24	I	O	C	O	O	O	O	I	1	O	O	C
methylprednisolone	O	O	6	24	O	O	I	O	O	O	O	I	C	O	24	O
mezlocillin	O	I	O	O	O	O	O	O	O	O	O	O	O	O	O	O
moxalactam	O	O	O	O	O	O	O	O	O	O	O	O	O	O	O	O
multiple vitamin infusion (MVI)	O	O	O	C	O	O	C	O	O	C	24	O	O	O	24	O
nafcillin	O	O	12	O	I	O	O	O	I	I	I	I	I	O	O	O
netilmicin	O	O	O	O	O	O	O	O	I	I	I	I	I	I	I	O
norepinephrine (levarterenol)	O	24	I	24	O	O	C	O	O	O	O	I	O	O	O	C
0.9% NSS	C	24	C	C	8	C	C	C	C	C	C	C	C	C	C	C
oxacillin	O	8	I	24	I	O	O	O	O	O	O	I	I	O	O	O
oxytocin	O	O	O	O	O	O	O	O	O	O	O	O	O	O	O	O
penicillin G	O	8	I	24	I	O	C	O	O	C	O	I	C	24	24	C
phytonadione	O	24	I	24	I	O	O	O	O	O	O	I	C	O	O	O
piperacillin	O	I	O	O	O	O	O	O	O	O	O	O	O	O	O	O
polymyxin B	O	24	O	O	I	O	I	I	O	I	O	I	I	O	O	O
potassium chloride	O	4	C	24	C	C	C	24	O	C	O	C	C	24	24	C
procainamide	O	I	C	O	C	O	C	O	O	O	O	O	C	O	O	C
sodium bicarbonate	O	24	C	O	I	C	I	24	O	O	24	C	C	C	24	I
tetracycline	O	8	I	24	I	O	I	I	O	I	O	I	I	O	O	C
thiamine	O	O	O	O	O	O	O	O	O	O	O	O	O	O	O	O
ticarcillin	O	I	O	O	I	O	O	O	O	O	O	O	O	O	O	O
tobramycin	O	O	O	O	O	O	I	I	I	I	I	I	O	O	I	O
vancomycin	O	24	I	O	O	O	I	I	O	O	O	O	I	O	O	C
verapamil	O	O	C	O	C	C	O	O	O	O	O	O	O	O	O	O
vitamin B complex with C	O	24	I	O	I	O	C	I	O	C	24	C	I	24	24	O

126 DRUG INTERACTIONS

DRUG INTERACTIONS

APPENDIX

COMBINATION DRUG PRODUCTS

Each drug product listed below is a combination of at least two drugs. If your patient's taking one of these combination products, check the list to identify the drugs contained in the product. Before administering another drug to the patient, consider whether an interaction is likely to occur.

Note: The products listed here are prescription products available only in the United States, unless otherwise noted.

ANTIDEPRESSANTS

Limbitrol 5-12.5: chlordiazepoxide 5 mg and amitriptyline (as HCl) 12.5 mg.
Limbitrol 10-25: chlordiazepoxide 10 mg and amitriptyline (as HCl) 25 mg.
Triavil-2-10, Triavil-2-25, Triavil-4-10, and Triavil-4-25 are products identical to the Etrafon products listed below. Triavil is also available as Triavil-4-50 (perphenazine 4 mg and amitriptyline HCl 50 mg).

Available in the United States and Canada:
Etrafon: perphenazine 2 mg and amitriptyline HCl 25 mg.
Etrafon 2-10: perphenazine 2 mg and amitriptyline HCl 10 mg.
Etrafon-A: perphenazine 4 mg and amitriptyline 10 mg.
Etrafon-Forte: perphenazine 4 mg and amitriptyline 25 mg.

ANTIFUNGALS

Achrostatin-V: nystatin 250,000 units and tetracycline HCl 250 mg.
Declostatin Caps: nystatin 250,000 units and demeclocycline HCl 150 mg.
Declostatin Tabs: nystatin 500,000 units and demeclocycline HCL 300 mg.
Mysteclin-F Caps: tetracycline HCl 250 mg and amphotericin B 50 mg, buffered with potassium metaphosphate.
Mysteclin-F Syrup: tetracycline HCl 125 mg and amphotericin B 25 mg/ml, buffered with potassium metaphosphate.
Terrastatin Caps: nystatin 250,000 units and oxytetracycline 250 mg.
Tetrastatin Caps: nystatin 250,000 units and tetracycline HCl 250 mg.

ANTIHYPERTENSIVES

Aldoclor-150: chlorothiazide 150 mg and methyldopa 250 mg.
Aldoclor-250: chlorothiazide 250 mg and methyldopa 250 mg.
Aldoril D30: hydrochlorothiazide 30 mg and methyldopa 500 mg.
Aldoril D50: hydrochlorothiazide 50 mg and methyldopa 500 mg.
Apresazide 25/25: hydrochlorothiazide 25 mg and hydralazine HCl 25 mg.
Apresazide 50/50: hydrochlorothiazide 50 mg and hydralazine HCl 50 mg.
Apresazide 100/50: hydrochlorothiazide 50 mg and hydralazine HCl 100 mg.
Apresoline-Esidrix: hydrochlorothiazide 15 mg and hydralazine HCl 25 mg.
Combipres 0.2: chlorthalidone 15 mg and clonidine HCl 0.2 mg.
Demi-Regroton: chlorthalidone 25 mg and reserpine 0.125 mg.
Diupres-250: chlorothiazide 250 mg and reserpine 0.125 mg.
Diupres-500: chlorothiazide 500 mg and reserpine 0.125 mg.
Diutensen: methyclothiazide 2.5 mg and cryptenamine 2 mg (as tannate).
Diutensen-R: methyclothiazide 2.5 mg and reserpine 0.1 mg.
Enduronyl: methyclothiazide 5 mg and deserpidine 0.25 mg.
Enduronyl-Forte: methyclothiazide 5 mg and deserpidine 0.5 mg.
Esimil. hydrochlorothiazide 25 mg and guanethidine monosulfate 10 mg.
Eutron Filmtabs: methyclothiazide 5 mg and pargyline HCl 25 mg.
Exna-R Tablets: benzthiazide 50 mg and reserpine 0.125 mg.
Hydromox-R: quinethazone 50 mg and reserpine 0.125 mg.
Hydroserp: hydrochlorothiazide 50 mg and reserpine 0.125 mg.
Hydrotensin-25 Tablets: hydrochlorothiazide 25 mg and reserpine 0.125 mg.
Hydrotensin-50: hydrochlorothiazide 50 mg and reserpine 0.125 mg.
Inderide 40/25: propranolol HCl 40 mg and hydrochlorothiazide 25 mg.
Inderide 80/25: propranolol HCl 80 mg and hydrochlorothiazide 25 mg.
Metatensin Tablets: trichlormethiazide 2 or 4 mg and reserpine 0.1 mg.
Naquival: trichlormethiazide 4 mg and reserpine 0.1 mg.
Oreticyl 25: hydrochlorothiazide 25 mg and deserpidine 0.125 mg.
Oreticyl 50: hydrochlorothiazide 50 mg and deserpidine 0.125 mg.
Oreticyl Forte: hydrochlorothiazide 25 mg and deserpidine 0.25 mg.
Rautrax: flumethiazide 400 mg, potassium chloride 400 mg, and powdered rauwolfia serpentina 50 mg. (May also contain tartrazine.)
Rautrax-N: bendroflumethiazide 4 mg, powdered rauwolfia ser-

pentina 50 mg, and potassium chloride 400 mg. (May also contain tartrazine.)
Rauzide: bendroflumethiazide 4 mg and powdered rauwolfia serpentina 50 mg. (May also contain tartrazine.)
Regroton: chlorthalidone 50 mg and reserpine 0.25 mg.
Renese-R: polythiazide 2 mg and reserpine 0.25 mg.
Salutensin-Demi: hydroflumethiazide 25 mg and reserpine 0.125 mg.
Serpasil-Apresoline #1: reserpine 0.1 mg and hydralazine HCl 25 mg.
Timolide 10/25: timolol maleate 10 mg and hydrochlorothiazide 25 mg.
Unipres: hydrochlorothiazide 15 mg, reserpine 0.1 mg, and hydralazine HCl 25 mg.

Available in the United States and Canada:
Aldoril-15: hydrochlorothiazide 15 mg and methyldopa 250 mg.
Aldoril-25: hydrochlorothiazide 25 mg and methyldopa 250 mg.
Combipres 0.1: chlorthalidone 15 mg and clonidine HCl 0.1 mg.
Hydropres-25: hydrochlorothiazide 25 mg and reserpine 0.125 mg.
Hydropres-50: hydrochlorothiazide 50 mg and reserpine 0.125 mg.
Naturetin W/K 2.5 mg: bendroflumethiazide 2.5 mg and potassium chloride 500 mg.
Naturetin W/K 5 mg: bendroflumethiazide 5 mg and potassium chloride 500 mg.
Salutensin: hydroflumethiazide 50 mg and reserpine 0.125 mg.
Ser-Ap-Es: hydrochlorothiazide 15 mg, reserpine 0.1 mg, and hydralazine HCl 25 mg.

Serpasil-Apresoline #2: reserpine 0.2 mg and hydralazine HCl 50 mg.
Serpasil-Esidrix #1 (called Serpasil-Esidrix 25 in Canada): hydrochlorothiazide 25 mg and reserpine 0.1 mg.
Serpasil-Esidrix #2 (called Serpasil-Esidrix 50 in Canada): hydrochlorothiazide 50 mg and reserpine 0.1 mg.

ANTIPSYCHOTICS

Triavil 2-10, Triavil 2-25, Triavil-4-10, and Triavil 4-25 are products identical to Etrafon products listed below; Triavil 4-50: perphenazine 4 mg and amitriptyline HCl 50 mg.

Available in the United States and Canada:
Etrafon 2-10: perphenazine 2 mg and amitripyline HCl 10 mg.
Etrafon-A: perphenazine 4 mg and amitriptyline 10 mg.
Etrafon-Forte: perphenazine 4 mg and amitriptyline 25 mg.

ANTITUBERCULARS

Rifamate: isoniazid 150 mg and rifampin 300 mg.
Teebaconin with vitamin B_6: isoniazid 100 mg and pyridoxine HCl 10 mg.

NARCOTIC AND OPIOID ANALGESICS

Empirin with codeine No. 2: aspirin 325 mg and codeine phosphate 15 mg.
Empirin with codeine No. 3: aspirin 325 mg and codeine phosphate 30 mg.
Empirin with codeine No. 4: aspirin 325 mg and codeine phosphate 60 mg.
Fiorinal with codeine No. 1: butalbital 50 mg, caffeine 40 mg, aspirin 325 mg, and codeine phosphate 7.5 mg.
Fiorinal with codeine No. 2: butalbital 50 mg, caffeine 40 mg, aspirin 200 mg, codeine phosphate 15 mg.
Fiorinal with codeine No. 3: butalbital 50 mg, caffeine 40 mg, aspirin 200 mg, and codeine phosphate 30 mg.
Percocet-5: acetaminophen 325 mg and oxycodone hydrochloride 5 mg.
Talacen: pentazocine hydrochloride 25 mg and acetaminophen 650 mg.
Tylox: acetaminophen 500 mg, oxycodone hydrochloride 4.5 mg, and oxycodone terephthalate 0.38 mg.

Available in the United States and Canada:
Innovar (Injection): fentanyl (as citrate) 0.05 mg and droperidol 2.5 mg/ml.
Pantopon: hydrochlorides of opium alkaloids (20 mg is therapeutically equivalent to 15 mg morphine).
Percodan: oxycodone hydrochloride 4.5 mg, oxycodone terephthalate 0.38 mg, and aspirin 325 mg.
Percodan-Demi: oxycodone hydrochloride 2.25 mg, oxycodone terephthalate 0.19 mg, and aspirin 325 mg.
Tylenol with codeine No. 1: acetaminophen 300 mg and codeine phosphate 7.5 mg.
Tylenol with codeine No. 2: acetaminophen 300 mg and codeine phosphate 15 mg.
Tylenol with codeine No. 3: acetaminophen 300 mg and codeine phosphate 30 mg.
Tylenol with codeine No. 4: acetaminophen 300 mg and codeine phosphate 60 mg.

Note: In Canada, all Tylenol with codeine products contain caffeine 15 mg.

CONTINUED ON PAGE 130

APPENDIX

COMBINATION DRUG PRODUCTS CONTINUED

NONNARCOTIC ANALGESICS AND ANTIPYRETICS

Alka-Seltzer Effervescent Pain Reliever and Antacid (OTC): aspirin 324 mg, sodium 24 mEq, sodium bicarbonate 1.904 g, and citric acid 1 g.

Allerest Headache Strength (OTC): acetaminophen 325 mg, chlorpheniramine maleate 2 mg, and phenylpropanolamine hydrochloride 18.7 mg.

Anacin: aspirin 400 mg and caffeine 32 mg.

A.P.C.: aspirin 227 mg, phenacetin 162 mg, and caffeine 32 mg.

Arthritis Pain Formula (OTC): aspirin 486 mg, aluminum hydroxide 20 mg, and magnesium hydroxide 60 mg.

A.S.A. Compound: aspirin 227 mg, phenacetin 160 mg, and caffeine 32.5 mg.

Bayer Aspirin (OTC): aspirin 325 mg and sodium 3.2 mEq.

Bufferin (OTC): aspirin 324 mg, magnesium carbonate 97.2 mg, and aluminum glycinate 48.6 mg.

Bufferin—Arthritis Strength (OTC): aspirin 486 mg, magnesium carbonate 145.8 mg, and aluminum glycinate 72.9 mg.

Darvocet-N 50: acetaminophen 325 mg and propoxyphene napsylate 50 mg.

Darvocet-N 100: acetaminophen 650 mg and propoxyphene napsylate 100 mg.

Darvon Compound-65: propoxyphene HCl 65 mg, aspirin 389 mg, and caffeine 32.4 mg.

Doan's Pills (OTC): caffeine 32 mg and magnesium salicylate 325 mg.

Equagesic: aspirin 250 mg, ethoheptazine citrate 75 mg, and meprobamate 150 mg.

Excedrin: aspirin 250 mg, acetaminophen 250 mg, and caffeine 65 mg.

Excedrin P.M. (OTC): aspirin 250 mg, acetaminophen 250 mg, and pyrilamine maleate 25 mg.

Femcaps: acetaminophen 324 mg, caffeine 32 mg, ephedrine sulfate 8 mg, and atropine sulfate 0.0325 mg.

Fiorinal: butalbital 50 mg, aspirin 200 mg, phenacetin 130 mg, and caffeine 40 mg.

Gemnisyn (OTC): aspirin 325 mg and acetaminophen 325 mg.

Midol Caplets (OTC): aspirin 454 mg, caffeine 32.4 mg, and cinnamedrine HCl 14.9 mg.

Momentum (OTC): aspirin 162.5 mg, salicylsalicylic acid 325 mg, and phenyltoloxamine citrate 12.5 mg.

Pamprin (OTC): acetaminophen 325 mg, pamabrom 25 mg, and pyrilamine maleate 12.5 mg.

Pamprin—Maximum Cramp Relief Formula (OTC): acetaminophen 500 mg, pamabrom 25 mg, and pyrilamine maleate 15 mg.

Sinarest (Regular Strength) (OTC): acetaminophen 325 mg, phenylpropanolamine hydrochloride 18.7 mg, and chlorpheniramine maleate 2 mg. (Extra-Strength contains 500 mg of acetaminophen.)

Sine-Aid (OTC): acetaminophen 325 mg and phenylpropanolamine hydrochloride 25 mg.

Synalgos: promethazine HCl 6.25 mg, aspirin 194.4 mg, phenacetin 162 mg, and caffeine 30 mg.

Talwin Compound Caplets: aspirin 325 mg and pentazocine (as HCl) 12.5 mg.

Trigesic (OTC): aspirin 230 mg, acetaminophen 125 mg, and caffeine 30 mg.

Trilisate: choline salicylate 293 mg and magnesium salicylate 362 mg.

Vanquish: aspirin 227 mg, acetaminophen 194 mg, caffeine 33 mg, aluminum hydroxide 25 mg, and magnesium hydroxide 50 mg.

Zactirin: aspirin 325 mg and ethoheptazine citrate 75 mg.

SEDATIVES AND HYPNOTICS

Carbrital Kapseals: pentobarbital sodium 97.5 mg and carbromal 260 mg.

Tri-Barbs Capsules: phenobarbital 32 mg, butabarbital sodium 32 mg, and secobarbital sodium 32 mg.

Tuinal 50 mg Pulvules: amobarbital sodium 25 mg and secobarbital sodium 25 mg.

Available in the United States and Canada:

Tuinal 100 mg Pulvules: amobarbital sodium 50 mg and secobarbital sodium 50 mg.

SULFONAMIDES

Azo Gantanol: sulfamethoxazole 500 mg and phenazopyridine hydrochloride 100 mg.

Azo Gantrisin: sulfisoxazole 500 mg and phenazopyridine hydrochloride 50 mg.

Azotrex: sulfamethizole 250 mg, tetracycline phosphate complex equivalent to 125 mg tetracycline HCl activity, and phenazopyridine hydrochloride 50 mg.

Suladyne: sulfamethizole 125 mg, sulfadiazine 125 mg, and phenazopyridine hydrochloride 75 mg.

Thiosulfil-A: sulfamethizole 250 mg and phenazopyridine hydrochloride 50 mg.

Triple Sulfa: sulfadiazine 167 mg, sulfamerazine 167 mg, and sulfamethazine 167 mg.

Urobiotic-250: sulfamethizole 250 mg, oxytetracycline (as HCl) 250 mg, and phenazopyridine hydrochloride 50 mg.

REFERENCES AND ACKNOWLEDGMENTS

Books

Abrams, Anne C. *Clinical Drug Therapy: Rationales for Nursing Practice.* Philadelphia: J.B. Lippincott Co., 1983.

AMA Drug Evaluations, 5th ed. Prepared by the AMA Division of Drugs. Chicago: American Medical Association, 1983.

Avery, Graeme S. *Drug Treatment: Principles and Practice of Clinical Pharmacology*, 2nd ed. Sydney: Australasian Drug Information Services (Division of ADIS Press), 1980.

Brunner, Lillian S., and Suddarth, Doris. *The Lippincott Manual of Nursing Practice*, 3rd ed. Philadelphia: J.B. Lippincott Co., 1982.

Drug Information for the Health Care Provider, USPDI Vol. 1. Rockville, Md.: United States Pharmacopeial Convention, 1983.

Drug Interaction Facts. St. Louis: J.B. Lippincott Co. (Facts and Comparisons Division).

Drugs, 2nd ed. Nurse's Reference Library. Springhouse, Pa.: Springhouse Corp., 1984.

Evaluations of Drug Interactions: 1976. Washington, D.C.: American Pharmaceutical Association, 1976.

Goodman, Louis S., and Gilman, Alfred, eds. *Goodman and Gilman's The Pharmacological Basis of Therapeutics*, 6th ed. New York: Macmillan Publishing Co., 1980.

Govoni, Laura E., and Hayes, Janice E. *Drugs and Nursing Implications*, 4th ed. East Norwalk, Conn.: Appleton-Century-Crofts, 1983.

Hansten, Philip D. *Drug Interactions*, 4th ed. Philadelphia: Lea & Febiger, 1979.

Knoben, James, E., and Anderson, Philip O., eds. *Handbook of Clinical Drug Data*, 5th ed. Hamilton, Ill.: Drug Intelligence Publications, 1983.

Martin, Eric W. *Hazards of Medication*, 2nd ed. New York: Harper & Row Publishers, 1978.

McEvoy, Gerald K., ed. *American Hospital Formulary Service: Drug Information 1984.* Washington, D.C.: American Society of Hospital Pharmacists, 1984.

The Medical Letter on Drugs and Therapeutics. New Rochelle, N.Y.: The Medical Letter.

Nursing84 Drug Handbook. Springhouse, Pa.: Springhouse Corp., 1984.

Pagliaro, Louis A., and Pagliaro, Ann M., eds. *Pharmacologic Aspects of Aging.* St. Louis: C.V. Mosby Co., 1983.

Rayburn, William F. "Common Over-the-Counter Drugs and Illicit Drug Use" and "Perinatal Pharmacology and Medications During Pregnancy," in Zuspan, Frederick P., and Quillagan, Edward J. *Practical Manual of Obstetric Care: A Pocket Reference for Those Who Treat the Pregnant Patient.* St. Louis: C.V. Mosby Co., 1982.

Spencer, Roberta T., and Nichols, Lynn W. *Clinical Pharmacology and Nursing Management.* Philadelphia: J.B. Lippincott Co., 1983.

Stockley, Ivan H. *Drug Interaction.* St. Louis: C.V. Mosby Co., 1981.

Trissel, Lawrence A. *Handbook of Injectable Drugs*, 3rd ed. Washington, D.C.: American Society of Hospital Pharmacists, 1983.

Vaughan, Victor C. III, et. al. *Nelson Textbook of Pediatrics*, 12th ed. Philadelphia: W.B. Saunders Co., 1983.

Periodicals

Darovic, Gloria Oblouk. "Infarction or Something Else?" *RN* 47(2):48-9, February 1984.

Deglin, J.M., and Mandell, H.N. "Drug Interactions Without Anguish," *Postgraduate Medicine* 72:199-205, 1982.

Deglin, Judith M. "Protecting Your Patients From Drug Interactions," *NursingLife* 3(4):33-44, July/August 1983.

Hayes, A.H., Jr. "How Drugs Affect Drugs," *Emergency Medicine* 13:114-43, July 15, 1981.

Karas, Stephen, Jr. "The Potential for Drug Interactions," *Annals of Emergency Medicine* 10(12):627-30, December 1981.

Lehmann, Phyllis. "Foods You Eat Can Affect the Medications You Take," *Your Life and Health* 96:16-18, November 1981.

Manzo, Mark. "A Drug By Any Other Name: Your Guide to Generic and Brand Names," *Nursing83* 13(11):97-112, November 1983.

Poirier, Therese I. "Factors Involved in Adverse Drug Reactions," *U.S. Pharmacist* 8(4):33-52, April 1983.

Rodman, Morton J. "New Drugs of the Year: A Host of Major Breakthroughs...Calcium Channel Blockers, Potent Third-Generation Antibiotics, and...the First Antiviral Against Genital Herpes," Parts 1, 2. *RN* 46 (April, May 1983):63,69.

Sause, Robert B., and Chin, Thomas H. "OTC Drug-Drug Reactions," *Journal of Practical Nursing* 33(4):20-31, April 1983.

We'd like to thank the following people for their help with this book:

CLARA LEWIS, RD, MS
  Associate Professor of Nutrition
  University of North Carolina
  School of Nursing
  Chapel Hill

DAVID RODGERS, MD
  Chestnut Hill Hospital
  Philadelphia

INDEX

A

Absorption
  acids and bases and, 49
  drug complexes, 49
  gastrointestinal, 19-21
  in geriatrics, 69
  mechanisms of, 17-18
  in pediatrics, 67
  and pharmacokinetics, 17
  rate versus amount, 49
Acetaminophen
  effects on lab tests, 121
  with warfarin and dicumarol, 100
Acetazolamide, effects on lab tests, 121-122
Active transport, 18
Additive interactions, 16, 54
A.D.M.E., 48
Adverse reaction
  definition of, 16
  identifying, 31
  preventing, 29, 31-32
  versus a side effect, 29
Alcohol
  with anticonvulsants, 101
  with barbiturates, 116
  with cefoperazone, cefamandole, and moxalactam, 95
  with metronidazole, 97
  with oral antidiabetics, 103
  with phenothiazines and haloperidol, 117
  with phenytoin, 102
  with procarbazine, 105
  with warfarin and dicumarol, 98
Allergy
  definition of, 16
  desensitization, 37
  forming of an, 33-34
  identifying an, 34
  and topical drugs, 34
  versus idiosyncrasy, 35
Allopurinol
  with ampicillin, 95
  with azathioprine and mercaptopurine, 105
Aminoglutethimide, effects on lab tests, 124
Aminoglycosides, interactions affecting therapy, 93, 94
Aminophylline, effect on lab test, 121, 124
Aminosalicylic acid, effect on lab tests, 121
Amitriptyline, effect on urine color, 125
Amphetamines, effects on lab tests, 122
Amphetamines or amphetamine-like drugs, with guanethidine, 108
Amphotericin B
  with corticosteroids, 96, 113
  with diuretics, 96
Ampicillin, with allopurinol, 95

Analgesics, interactions affecting therapy, 91-92
Anaphylaxis
  definition of, 16
  how it develops, 35
  how to intervene, 36-37
Androgens
  effect on lab tests, 124
  with warfarin and dicumarol, 100
Antacids
  geriatric adverse reactions, 72
  interactions affecting therapy, 112
  with iron salts, 112
  with isoniazid, 97
  with phenothiazines and haloperidol, 117
  with salicylates, 91
  with tetracyclines, 96
Antagonistic interactions, 55
Anthraquinone laxative, effect on urine color, 125
Antianxiety agents, geriatric adverse reactions, 72
Antiarrhythmics, interactions affecting therapy, 106-107
Anticholinergics
  with digoxin, 111
  geriatric adverse reaction, 72
  with phenothiazines and haloperidol, 117
Anticonvulsants
  interactions affecting therapy, 101-102
  with phenothiazines and tricyclic antidepressants, 101
Antidiabetics, with dicumarol, 100
Antifungal agents, interactions affecting therapy, 93
Antifungals, combination drug products, 128
Antigen, definition of, 16
Antihistamines
  geriatric adverse reactions, 72
  pharmacogenetic reactions, 75
  and the pregnant patient, 64
Antihypertensives
  with calcium channel blockers, 110
  combination drug products, 128
  interactions affecting therapy, 107-109
  use with dialysis, 77
Anti-infectives
  interactions affecting therapy, 93-97
  use with dialysis, 77
  with warfarin, 93
Antimalarials, 74
Antineoplastics, interactions affecting therapy, 105
Antipsychotics, combination drug products, 129
Antipyretics, combination drug products, 130
Antituberculars, combination drug products, 129

Ascorbic acid
  effect on lab tests, 121
  how smoking affects, 86
Aspirin
  and the pregnant patient, 64
  with spironolactone, 111
Assessment
  arm measurement values, 11
  fat and protein reserves, 10
  kidney function, 76
  liver disease, 79-80
  liver function, 80-81
  special considerations, 9
Atypical pseudocholinesterase, drug reactions from, 74
Azathioprine, with allopurinol, 105

B

Barbiturate anesthetics, with narcotics, 92
Barbiturates
  administration of, 115
  with corticosteroids, 113
  effect on lab tests, 122
  geriatric adverse reactions, 72
  interactions affecting therapy, 116
  with metoprolol and propranolol, 109
  with oral contraceptives, 114
  with quinidine, 107
  with warfarin and dicumarol, 99
Barium sulfate, effects on lab tests, 121
Benzodiazepines, with cimetidine, 112
Beta adrenergic blockers
  with barbiturates, 116
  with calcium channel blockers, 110
  effect on lab tests, 122
  interactions affecting therapy, 109
  with lidocaine, 106
  with oral antidiabetics, 103
  with prazosin, 109
  use in cardiovascular drug therapy, 106
Binding-site competition, 49-50
Bioavailability
  definition of, 16
  understanding, 40
Bioequivalent, 16
Biotin, for fetal disorders, 65
Biotransformation, definition of, 16
Blood-brain barrier, 23
Body frame, determining, 9
Bretylium, effects on lab tests, 125
Bromsulphalein, methodologic interactions, 121
Bronchodilators, with beta adrenergic blockers, 109
Burns, effects on drug action, 83

C

Caffeine
  effects on lab tests, 124
  and the pregnant patient, 65

Calcium channel blockers
  interactions affecting therapy, 110
  therapeutic use of, 106
Calcium gluconate, effects on lab tests, 121
Calcium imbalances, 56-57
Captopril
  effects on lab tests, 121
  interactions affecting therapy, 108
Carbamazepine
  effects on lab tests, 121
  interactions affecting therapy, 101
  with isoniazid, 97
  therapeutic use of, 101
  with warfarin and dicumarol, 99
Carbonic anhydrase inhibitors
  with quinidine, 107
  with salicylates, 91
Cardiogenic shock, effects on drug action, 83
Cascara, effect on lab tests, 121, 125
Cathartics, use with dialysis, 77
Cefamandole, with alcohol, 95
Cefoperazone, with alcohol, 95
Cephalosporins
  effects on lab tests, 121
  interactions affecting therapy, 93
  with probenecid, 95
Cephalothin, with aminoglycosides, 94
Chloral hydrate
  effects on lab tests, 121
  with warfarin and dicumarol, 99
Chloramphenicol
  with oral antidiabetics, 103
  with phenytoin, 102
  with vitamin B_{12}, 119
Chlordiazepoxide, how smoking affects, 86
Chloroquine, effect on urine color, 125
Chlorpromazine
  geriatric adverse reactions, 72
  how smoking affects, 86
  with meperidine, 92
  with metoprolol and propranolol, 109
Chlorzoxazone, effect on urine color, 125
Cholestyramine
  with digitoxin, 111
  with thyroid hormones, 114
  with warfarin and dicumarol, 99
Cimetidine
  with benzodiazepines and theophylline, 112
  geriatric adverse reaction, 72
  with lidocaine, 106
  with narcotics, 92
  with phenytoin, 102
  with propranolol, 109
  with quinidine, 107
  with warfarin and dicumarol, 100
Clofibrate
  effects on lab tests, 122
  with warfarin and dicumarol, 99

Clonidine
  effects on lab tests, 124
  with levodopa and tricyclic antidepressants, 108
Coffee, effect on lab tests, 121
Colestipol
  with digitoxin, 111
  with thyroid hormones, 114
  with warfarin and dicumarol, 99
Combination drug products, 128-130
Competitive binding
  and distribution, 49-50
  drug displacers, 51
Contrast media containing iodine, effects on lab tests, 121, 124
Corticosteroids
  with amphotericin B, 96
  with barbiturates, 116
  with diuretics, 111
  effect on lab tests, 122, 124
  interactions affecting therapy, 113
  with isoniazid, 97
  with salicylates, 91

D

Danthron, effect on lab tests, 121, 125
Dapsone, 74
Daunorubicin, effect on urine color, 125
Deferoxamine, effect on urine color, 125
Desensitization, 37
Dextran, effects on lab tests, 121
Dialysis, drugs and, 77
Dialyzable drugs, 78
Diazepam, how smoking affects, 86
Diazoxide, effects on lab tests, 122, 123
Dicumarol
  interactions affecting therapy, 98-100
  with oral antidiabetics, 104
Digitalis glycosides
  with corticosteroids, 113
  effects on lab tests, 121
  interactions affecting therapy, 110-111
  with methimazole and propylthiouracil, 114
  use with dialysis, 77
Digitoxin, with cholestyramine and colestipol, 111
Digoxin
  with calcium channel blockers, 110
  for fetal disorders, 65
  geriatric adverse reactions, 72
  interactions affecting therapy, 111
Disopyramide
  with calcium channel blockers, 110
  with lidocaine, 106

Distribution
  blood-brain barrier, 23
  and competitive binding, 49-50
  drug displacers, 51
  in geriatrics, 69
  in pediatrics, 67
  protein binding, 22-23
  receptor sites, 21-22
Disulfiram
  with metronidazole, 97
  with phenytoin, 102
  with warfarin and dicumarol, 99
Diuretics
  with amphotericin B, 96
  with corticosteroids, 111
  effect on lab tests, 122, 123
  geriatric adverse reactions, 72
Diuretics, potassium-sparing. *See* Potassium-sparing diuretics. *See also* Loop diuretics *and* Thiazide diuretics.
Doxycycline, with barbiturates, 116
Drug administration
  comparing routes, 38-39
  considerations, 38
Drug complexes and absorption, 49
Drug half-life, 28
Drug history, 8
Drug interactions
  classifying, 46
  dealing with, 90
  effect on drug processing, 48-53
  identifying, 47
  specific, 91-119
Drug toxicity
  preventing, 31-32
  types of, 31-32

E

Electrolytes
  drug interactions with, 58
  effects of imbalances on drug therapy, 55-57
Enteric-coated drugs, with antacids, 112
Enzyme induction, definition of, 16
Epinephrine
  effects on lab tests, 122, 124, 125
  with tricyclic antidepressants, 115
Ergot alkaloids, effects on lab tests, 123
Erythromycin
  with carbamazepine, 101
  effects on lab tests, 121
  with theophylline, 93, 96
Estrogen, effect on lab tests, 121-123
Ethambutol, effect on lab tests, 124
Ethanol, effect on lab tests, 122
Ethinamate, effect on lab tests, 121
Ethoxazene, effect on urine color, 125

DRUG INTERACTIONS 133

INDEX

Excretion
  considerations, 26
  in geriatrics, 69
  interactions, 53
  by kidney, 26, 76
  in pediatrics, 67
  understanding, 26-28

F

Fat emulsion I.V., effects on lab tests, 121, 122
Fat reserves, assessing, 10
Fenfluramine, with oral antidiabetics, 104
Ferrous salts, effect on urine color, 125
Fetal
  circulation, 64
  drug action, 63
  drug therapy, 65
First-pass metabolism, 25
Fluorescein, effect on urine color, 125
Flurazepam, geriatric adverse reaction, 72
Folic acid
  with phenytoin, 102
  with sulfasalazine, 119
Food/drug interactions, 41, 86-87
Free drug, definition of, 16
Furazolidone, effect on urine color, 125
Furosemide, geriatric adverse reactions, 72

G

G6PD deficiency, 73-75
Gastrointestinal absorption. *See* Absorption.
Gastrointestinal anticholinergics, with tricyclic antidepressants, 116
Gastrointestinal drugs, interactions affecting therapy, 112
Gastrointestinal pH, 21
Generic drugs, definition of, 16
Genetic deficiencies, drugs and, 72-75
Geriatrics
  drug action in, 69-70
  drug use, 71
  patient compliance, 70
  recognizing adverse reactions, 72
Glucocorticoids, for fetal disorders, 65
Glutethimide, with warfarin and dicumarol, 99
Guaifenesin, effect on lab tests, 121
Guanethidine, interactions affecting therapy, 108

H

Half-life, definition of, 16
Haloperidol
  effects on lab tests, 123
  with guanethidine, 108
  interactions affecting therapy, 117
Halothane, with ketamine, 119
Heparin, effects on lab tests, 121
Hepatic porphyria, 75
Hepatotoxicity, 82
Hormones
  how smoking affects, 86
  interactions affecting therapy, 113-114
Hydralazine, effect on lab tests, 121
Hydrochlorothiazide, geriatric adverse reaction, 72
Hypersensitivity, definition of, 16
Hypnotics
  combination drug products, 130
  geriatric adverse reactions, 72

I

Idiosyncrasy, 16, 35
Indomethacin
  effect on urine color, 125
  with lithium, 117
Inhalation anesthetics, 75
Inorganic iodides, effect on lab tests, 121
Insulin
  effect on lab tests, 124
  with MAO inhibitors, 118
Iopanoic acid, effect on lab tests, 122
Iron salts
  with antacids, 112
  with tetracyclines, 96
Iron sorbitex, effect on urine color, 125
Isoniazid
  interactions affecting therapy, 97
  with phenytoin, 102
Isopropamide, effect on lab tests, 121
Isoproterenol, effects on lab tests, 124

K

Ketamine, with halothane and tubocurarine, 119
Kidney disease, drugs and, 76-77
Kidneys
  assessing function of, 76
  drugs excreted by, 76
  reviewing function, 27
  role in drug excretion, 26

L

Lab tests
  drugs affecting test results, 120
  methodologic interactions, 121
  pharmacologic interactions, 122-125

Laxatives, and the pregnant patient, 65
Levodopa
  with clonidine, 108
  effects on lab tests, 121, 123, 125
  with MAO inhibitors, 118
  with phenytoin, 102
  with vitamin B_6, 119
Lidocaine, interactions affecting therapy, 106
Lithium
  administration considerations, 115
  effect on lab tests, 123
  interactions affecting therapy, 117-118
Liver
  assessing function of the, 80-81
  reviewing function of the, 24
Liver disease
  drugs and, 79
  effects on drug action, 82
  hepatotoxicity, 82
  planning drug therapy, 81-82
Loop diuretics, with aminoglycosides, 94

M

Magnesium imbalances, 56
Marijuana, effect on drug action, 84
Meperidine, interactions affecting therapy, 92
Mepivacaine, 75
Meprobamate, effects on lab tests, 121
Mercaptopurine, with allopurinol, 105
Metabolism
  first-pass, 25
  in geriatrics, 69
  interactions, 51-52
  liver function, 24
  in pediatrics, 67-68
  understanding, 24
  using enzyme inhibition and induction, 52
Metabolite, definition of, 16
Methadone, effect on lab tests, 123
Methenamine, effect on lab tests, 121
Methimazole, with digitalis glycosides, 114
Methocarbamol
  effect on urine color, 125
  effects on lab tests, 121
Methotrexate
  effects on lab tests, 124
  with salicylates and probenecid, 105
Methyldopa
  effects on lab tests, 121, 123-125
  geriatric adverse reaction, 72
  with lithium, 117
Methylene blue, effect on urine color, 125
Metoclopramide
  with digoxin, 111
  effects on lab tests, 123

Metoprolol, with chlorpromazine and barbiturates, 109
Metronidazole
　with alcohol and disulfiram, 97
　effect on urine color, 125
　with warfarin and dicumarol, 100
Mitotane, effect on lab tests, 125
Monoamine oxidase (MAO) inhibitors
　administration considerations, 115
　effects on lab tests, 123
　interactions affecting therapy, 118
　with meperidine, 92
　with oral antidiabetics, 104
　with tricyclic antidepressants, 115
Moxalactam, with alcohol, 95
Mydriatics, 75

N

Nalidixic acid, effect on lab tests, 121
Naproxen, effect on lab tests, 121
Narcotic analgesics
　combination drug products, 129
　geriatric adverse reaction, 72
　interactions affecting therapy, 92
Nephrotoxic drugs, 79, 124
Neuromuscular blocker agents
　with aminoglycosides, 94
　with lidocaine, 106
　with quinidine, 107
Nicotine
　effect on drug action, 84
　effect on lab tests, 122
Nitrates, with antihypertensives, 107
Nitrofurantoin, effect on urine color, 125
Nitroglycerin, effects on lab tests, 125
Nonnarcotic analgesics, combination drug products, 130
Nonsteroidal anti-inflammatory agents
　with captopril, 108
　with corticosteroids, 113
Nonsulfonamide antibacterial agents, 74
Norepinephrine, with tricyclic antidepressants, 115
Novobiocin, effects on lab tests, 122
Nutrition, how drugs affect, 87

O

Opioid analgesics
　combination drug products, 129
　interactions affecting therapy, 92
Oral anticoagulants, interactions affecting therapy, 98-100
Oral antidiabetics, interactions affecting therapy, 103-104
Oral contraceptives
　with barbiturates, 116
　effect on lab tests, 123, 125
　how smoking affects, 86
　interactions affecting therapy, 114

Oxyphenbutazone
　with oral antidiabetics, 103
　with phenytoin, 102
　with warfarin and dicumarol, 99

P

Para-aminosalicylic acid
　effect on lab tests, 123
　with vitamin B_{12}, 119
Passive diffusion, 17-18
Patient teaching, 11-12
Pediatrics, drug action in, 67-68
Penicillins
　with aminoglycosides, 94
　effects on lab tests, 121
　for fetal disorders, 65
　interaction affecting therapy, 93
　with probenecid, 95
　with tetracyclines, 96
Pentobarbital, geriatric adverse reactions, 72
Pharmacogenetic reactions, recognizing, 74-75
Phenazopyridine, effect on lab tests, 121, 125
Phenelzine, 74
Phenindione, effect on urine color, 125
Phenobarbital
　with carbamazepine, 101
　with valproic acid, 101
Phenolphthalein, effect on lab tests, 121, 125
Phenothiazines
　with anticonvulsants, 101
　with antihypertensives, 107
　effect on lab tests, 121, 123, 125
　with guanethidine, 108
　interactions affecting therapy, 117
Phensuximide, effect on urine color, 125
Phenylbutazone
　with oral antidiabetics, 103
　with phenytoin, 102
　with warfarin and dicumarol, 99
Phenytoin
　with corticosteroids, 113
　with dicumarol, 100
　effect on lab tests, 123, 125
　geriatric adverse reaction, 72
　interactions affecting therapy, 102
　with lidocaine, 106
　with meperidine, 92
　with quinidine, 107
　therapeutic use of, 101
Plasma cortisol
　methodologic interactions, 121
　pharmacologic interactions, 122
Potassium
　with captopril, 108
　imbalances, 55-56
　neuromuscular impulses, 57
Potassium-losing diuretics, interaction with lithium, 117

Potassium-sparing diuretics
　with captopril, 108
　interaction affecting therapy, 111
Potassium supplements, with potassium-sparing diuretics, 111
Potassium-wasting diuretics
　with corticosteroids, 113
　with digitalis glycosides, 110
Prazosin, with beta blockers, 109
Pregnancy
　drugs and, 62
　drugs and breast-feeding, 66
　drugs and the neonate, 65
　maternal drug action, 62-63
　over-the-counter drugs and, 64
Primaquine, effect on urine color, 125
Probenecid
　with cephalosporins, 95
　effects on lab tests, 125
　with methotrexate, 105
　with penicillins, 95
　with salicylates, 91
Procainamide, 74
Procarbazine, with alcohol, 105
Propoxyphene hydrochloride
　with carbamazepine, 101
　how smoking affects, 86
　interactions affecting therapy, 92
Propranolol
　how smoking affects, 86
　interactions affecting therapy, 109
Propylthiouracil, with digitalis glycosides, 114
Protein binding, 17, 22-23
Psychotherapeutic drugs
　how smoking affects, 86
　interactions affecting therapy, 115-118
Pyrazinamide, effects on lab tests, 124

Q

Quinacrine, effect on urine color, 125
Quinidine
　with barbiturates, 116
　with digoxin, 111
　effects on lab tests, 121
　geriatric adverse reactions, 72
　interactions affecting therapy, 107
　with warfarin and dicumarol, 99
Quinine, effect on lab tests, 121, 125

R

Receptor sites
　action, 54-55
　definition of, 21-22
Renal failure, 76
Reserpine
　effects on lab tests, 121
　geriatric adverse reaction, 72
Resorcinol, effect on urine color, 125
Respiratory failure, effects on drug action, 83
Riboflavin, effect on urine color, 125

INDEX

Rifampin
  with corticosteroids, 113
  effect on lab tests, 122, 125
  with oral antidiabetics, 104
  with oral contraceptives, 114
  with quinidine, 107
  with warfarin and dicumarol, 99

S

Salicylates
  with corticosteroids, 113
  effects on lab tests, 121, 122, 124
  interactions affecting therapy, 91
  with methotrexate, 105
  with warfarin, 91
  with warfarin and dicumarol, 98
Scopolamine, 75
Sedatives
  combination drug products, 130
  and the pregnant patient, 65
Senna, effect on urine color, 125
Serum bilirubin
  methodologic interactions, 121
  pharmacologic interactions, 122
Serum gamma glutamyl transpeptidase (GGT), pharmacologic interactions, 122
Serum glucose
  methodologic interactions, 121
  pharmacologic interactions, 122
Serum glutamic-pyruvic transaminase (SGPT), 80-81
Serum magnesium, methodologic interactions, 121
Serum prolactin, pharmacologic interactions, 123
Serum uric acid
  methodologic interactions, 121
  pharmacologic interactions, 123-124
Side effect, definition of, 17
Slow acetylator, 74
Smoking
  drug action and, 84
  effects on drug action, 86
  pregnancy and, 85
Sodium bicarbonate, effects on lab tests, 121
Sodium levothyroxine, 65
Spironolactone
  with aspirin, 111
  effect on lab tests, 121
Streptokinase, effects on lab tests, 122
Succinylcholine, 74
Sulfasalazine
  effect on urine color, 125
  with folic acid, 119
Sulfinpyrazone, with salicylates, 91

Sulfonamides
  combination drug products, 130
  effect on lab tests, 121, 125
  interactions affecting therapy, 93
  with oral antidiabetics, 104
  with phenytoin, 102
  with warfarin and dicumarol, 100
Sympathomimetics
  with guanethidine, 108
  with MAO inhibitors, 118
Synergistic interactions, 54

T

Testolactone, effects on lab tests, 125
Tetracyclines
  effects on lab tests, 121
  interactions affecting therapy, 93, 96
Theophylline
  with beta blockers, 109
  with cimetidine, 112
  with erythromycin, 93, 96
  how smoking affects, 86
  with oral contraceptives, 114
Therapeutic index, definition of, 17, 29
Thiazide diuretics, with oral antidiabetics, 104
Thiothixene, effects on lab tests, 123
Thyroid function
  methodologic interactions, 121
  pharmacologic interactions, 123
Thyroid hormone antagonists, with digitalis glycosides, 114
Thyroid hormones
  with cholestyramine or colestipol, 114
  with digitalis glycosides, 110
  with warfarin and dicumarol, 99
Tolbutamide, effects on lab tests, 121
Tolerance, 17, 32
Tolmetin, effects on lab tests, 121
Trauma, effects on drug action, 83
Triamterene, effect on urine color, 125
Tricyclic antidepressants
  administration considerations, 115
  with anticonvulsants, 101
  with clonidine, 108
  geriatric adverse reaction, 72
  with guanethidine, 108
  interactions affecting therapy, 115-116
  with MAO inhibitors, 118
Trimethoprim, with phenytoin, 102
Tubocurarine, with ketamine, 119

U

Urinary alkalinizers, with lithium, 118
Urine catecholamines
  methodologic interactions, 121
  pharmacologic interactions, 124
Urine color, drugs that affect, 125

Urine 5-hydroxyindoleacetic acid (5-HIAA), methodologic interactions, 121
Urine ketones, methodologic interactions, 121
Urine phenolsulfonphthalein (PSP), methodologic interactions, 121
Urine phenolsulfonphthalein (PSP) test, 120
Urine protein
  methodologic interactions, 121
  pharmacologic interactions, 124
Urine steroids
  methodologic interactions, 121
  pharmacologic interactions, 124-125
Urine testing, 76
Urine vanillylmandelic acid (VMA)
  methodologic interactions, 121
  pharmacologic interactions, 125

V

Valproic acid
  effects on lab tests, 121
  with phenobarbital, 101
  with phenytoin, 102
Vasopressin, effects on lab tests, 122
Vitamin B complex, effects on lab tests, 121
Vitamin B_6, with levodopa, 119
Vitamin B_{12}, with para-aminosalicylic acid and chloramphenicol, 119
Vitamin C, with quinidine, 107
Vitamin K, with anticoagulants, 98
Vitamins
  how smoking affects, 86
  and the pregnant patient, 64-65
  use with dialysis, 77

W

Warfarin, 75
  effect on urine color, 125
  interactions affecting therapy, 98-100
  with orally administered anti-infectives, 93
  with salicylates, 91, 98